THE AIP DIET COOKBOOK FOR BEGINNERS

Simple and Nutrient_Dense Recipes for the Relief of Autoimmune protocol Conditions

Jennifer Stewart

INTRODUCTION

Understanding the Autoimmune Protocol (AIP)

What is the AIP?

As a beginner, you might be wondering what exactly this diet is all about. In simple terms, the AIP diet is a way of eating that's designed to help people with autoimmune diseases feel better. Autoimmune diseases are conditions where the immune system, which is supposed to protect your body from harmful invaders, gets confused and starts attacking your own healthy cells. Imagine your immune system as a well-trained guard dog. Usually, it knows to attack only intruders, like bacteria or viruses. But sometimes, it gets confused and starts attacking its own family members—your body's healthy cells. This confusion leads to autoimmune diseases, which can cause symptoms like chronic pain, fatigue, and inflammation.

The AIP diet is like a retraining program for your immune system. It involves removing foods that can trigger inflammation and replacing them with nutrient-rich, healing foods. The goal is to calm down the immune response, reduce inflammation, and help your body heal.

History and Background of the AIP Diet

The concept of using diet to manage autoimmune diseases isn't new, but the AIP diet as we know it today has been shaped by recent scientific research and the experiences of people living with these conditions. It's based on the Paleo diet, which focuses on eating like our ancestors did—lots of fresh vegetables, fruits, meats, and fish, while avoiding processed foods, grains, dairy, and legumes.

Over time, experts noticed that some people with autoimmune diseases needed to take things a step further. They started identifying specific foods that seemed to trigger symptoms in many individuals and developed the AIP diet as a more targeted approach. It's a more restrictive version of Paleo, but it's all for a good reason, which is to help you feel your best.

Benefits of the AIP Diet for Autoimmune Conditions

So, why go through the trouble of following the AIP diet? The benefits can be life-changing. Here are some of the major perks:

1. Reduced Inflammation: Many people with autoimmune diseases struggle with chronic inflammation. The AIP diet eliminates foods known to cause inflammation, helping to soothe and calm the immune system.

2. Symptom Relief: Whether you're dealing with joint pain, digestive issues, skin problems, or fatigue, the AIP diet can help alleviate these symptoms by addressing the root cause.

3. Gut Health: A huge part of the AIP diet focuses on improving gut health. A healthy gut is crucial for a well-functioning immune system. By avoiding irritating foods and including gut-healing ones like bone broth and fermented vegetables, you're setting the stage for better overall health.

4. Nutrient Density: The AIP diet is packed with nutrient-dense foods. This means you're getting more vitamins, minerals, and antioxidants that your body needs to repair and thrive.

5. Personalized Health Insights: One of the great things about the AIP diet is that it's a journey of discovery. By systematically reintroducing foods, you can identify which ones are your personal triggers and tailor your diet to suit your unique needs.

Scientific Evidence Supporting the AIP Diet

You might be thinking, "This all sounds great, but does it really work?" The answer is yes, and there's growing scientific evidence to back it up. Studies have shown that the AIP diet can lead to significant improvements in symptoms and quality of life for people with various autoimmune diseases.

For example, a study published in 2017 found that people with inflammatory bowel disease (IBD) who followed the AIP diet experienced significant reductions in disease activity and improvements in quality of life. Another study in 2019 showed that individuals with Hashimoto's thyroiditis saw improvements in inflammation and symptoms after following the AIP diet.

While more research is always welcome, these studies provide strong support for what many people with autoimmune diseases have already discovered firsthand: the AIP diet can be a powerful tool in managing and improving their health.

Embarking on the AIP journey can feel overwhelming, but it doesn't have to be. The key is to take it one step at a time. Start by gradually eliminating the foods that can cause inflammation and stocking your kitchen with AIP-friendly alternatives. There are plenty of delicious and satisfying recipes to keep you nourished and satisfied.

Remember, the AIP diet is not about perfection but about progress. Listen to your body, be patient with yourself, and know that you're taking important steps towards better health.

Chapter 1:

Getting Started with AIP

What to Eat and Avoid

Embarking on the Autoimmune Protocol (AIP) diet might feel like a big change, but with the right guidance, it can be a smooth transition towards better health. Let's break it down step by step.

Approved Foods List

First things first, let's talk about what you can eat on the AIP diet. The focus is on nutrient-dense, whole foods that support healing and reduce inflammation. Here's a list of foods that are not only allowed but encouraged:

1. **Vegetables:** Load up on a variety of veggies, especially leafy greens and colorful vegetables. Sweet potatoes, carrots, squash, and cruciferous veggies like broccoli and cauliflower are great choices.
2. **Fruits:** Most fruits are allowed, but it's best to enjoy them in moderation due to their sugar content. Berries, apples, and bananas are good options.
3. **Meats and Fish:** Focus on high-quality, unprocessed meats. Grass-fed beef, pasture-raised poultry, wild-caught fish, and organ meats are excellent. Avoid processed meats and opt for fresh, natural sources of protein.
4. **Healthy Fats:** Include healthy fats like olive oil, coconut oil, and avocado oil in your diet. Avocados, olives, and coconut products are also great sources.
5. **Herbs and Spices:** Fresh herbs and non-seed spices can add flavor to your meals. Think garlic, ginger, basil, and turmeric.
6. **Bone Broth:** This is a powerhouse for gut healing. Bone broth is rich in collagen and nutrients that support the immune system and gut health.

7. **Fermented Foods:** Foods like sauerkraut, kimchi (without non-compliant ingredients), and kombucha can support a healthy gut microbiome.

Foods to Eliminate and Why

To understand why certain foods are eliminated, it helps to know a bit about how they can impact the immune system and gut health. The AIP diet removes foods that are known to be inflammatory or potentially problematic for people with autoimmune conditions. Here's what to avoid and why:

1. **Grains:** This includes wheat, rice, oats, and corn. Grains contain proteins like gluten and lectins that can irritate the gut lining and trigger inflammation.
2. **Legumes:** Beans, lentils, peanuts, and soy are off-limits. They contain lectins and other compounds that can be hard to digest and may contribute to gut inflammation.
3. **Dairy:** All forms of dairy, including milk, cheese, yogurt, and butter, are excluded. Dairy can be inflammatory and is a common allergen that may affect the immune system.
4. **Nightshades:** This family includes tomatoes, potatoes, eggplants, and peppers. Nightshades contain alkaloids that can cause inflammation in some people.
5. **Nuts and Seeds:** Even though they are often considered healthy, nuts and seeds can be hard on the gut and trigger immune responses. This includes nut-based oils and butters.
6. **Processed Foods:** Anything processed or refined, including sugars, artificial sweeteners, and additives, should be avoided. These foods can trigger inflammation and are often nutrient-poor.
7. **Eggs:** Eggs are a common allergen and can contribute to gut permeability, so they're excluded during the elimination phase.

Reintroduction Phase: How to Do It

The AIP diet isn't meant to be permanent. Once you've followed the elimination phase for at least 30 days and have experienced some symptom relief, you can start the reintroduction phase. This phase helps you identify which foods might be causing your symptoms. Here's how to do it:

1. **Choose One Food to Reintroduce:** Start with a food you miss the most or think is least likely to cause a reaction. For example, you might start with egg yolks.
2. **Eat the Food in Small Amounts:** On day one, eat a small amount of the food (like a teaspoon of egg yolk). Wait 15 minutes. If you don't have a reaction, eat a bit more (like a tablespoon) and wait for a few hours. Finally, have a normal portion if there are no adverse reactions.
3. **Monitor for Reactions:** Over the next 3-7 days, watch for any symptoms such as digestive upset, joint pain, headaches, or skin issues. If you notice any symptoms, stop the reintroduction and return to the elimination phase.
4. **Keep a Food Diary:** Document what you reintroduce, how much you eat, and any symptoms you experience. This helps you track your body's responses and identify patterns.
5. **Proceed Slowly:** Only reintroduce one new food every 3-7 days. This slow pace helps you accurately pinpoint which foods are problematic.
6. **Reassess and Adjust:** Based on your reactions, decide whether to include or permanently eliminate each food. Some foods might be reintroduced successfully, while others might need to be avoided long-term.

By taking it step by step, you can identify which foods support your health and which ones you need to avoid. The reintroduction phase is a powerful tool for creating a personalized diet that helps you feel your best.

Pantry and Kitchen Essentials

Embarking on the AIP journey means making some changes in your kitchen. Stocking up on the right ingredients and tools can make the transition smoother and more enjoyable. Let's break down what you need to set up an AIP-friendly kitchen, the essential tools and gadgets that will make cooking easier, and some ingredient substitutions to keep your meals delicious.

Stocking an AIP-Friendly Kitchen

Creating an AIP-friendly pantry starts with understanding what ingredients you'll need to support your new way of eating. Here's a guide to stocking your kitchen with AIP-approved items:

Pantry Staples:

1. **Oils and Fats:**
   - Coconut oil
   - Olive oil
   - Avocado oil
   - Lard or tallow (from grass-fed animals)
2. **Flours and Baking Ingredients:**
   - Coconut flour
   - Cassava flour
   - Arrowroot powder
   - Tigernut flour
3. **Broths and Stocks:**
   - Bone broth (homemade or store-bought without additives)
   - Fish stock
4. **Canned Goods:**
   - Coconut milk (full-fat, without additives)
   - Wild-caught tuna or salmon
5. **Sweeteners:**
   - Raw honey (in moderation)
   - Maple syrup (in moderation)
6. **Herbs and Spices:**
   - Fresh herbs (basil, thyme, rosemary, etc.)
   - Dried herbs (oregano, parsley, dill, etc.)
   - Turmeric, ginger, garlic powder

Fresh Produce:

1. Vegetables:
- Leafy greens (spinach, kale, Swiss chard)
- Cruciferous vegetables (broccoli, cauliflower, Brussels sprouts)
- Root vegetables (sweet potatoes, carrots, beets)
- Squashes (butternut, acorn, spaghetti)

2. Fruits:
- Berries (blueberries, strawberries, raspberries)
- Apples and pears
- Bananas
- Avocados

Proteins:

1. Meats:
- Grass-fed beef
- Pasture-raised poultry
- Wild-caught fish
- Organ meats (liver, heart, kidneys)

2. Others:
- Seafood (shrimp, scallops, crab)
- Eggs (if reintroduced)

Fermented Foods:

1. Probiotic-rich foods:
- Sauerkraut
- Kimchi (without non-compliant ingredients)
- Kombucha (watch for added sugars)

Essential Kitchen Tools and Gadgets

Having the right tools in your kitchen can make preparing AIP meals more efficient and enjoyable. Here are some essential gadgets and tools to consider:

1. **High-Quality Knife Set:** Invest in a good set of knives for chopping vegetables, fruits, and meats. A sharp chef's knife can make meal prep quicker and safer.
2. **Cutting Boards:** Use separate boards for meats and vegetables to avoid cross-contamination. Opt for sturdy wooden or plastic cutting boards.
3. **Food Processor:** A versatile tool for making cauliflower rice, chopping vegetables, and blending sauces or dips.
4. **Blender:** Essential for smoothies, soups, and sauces. A high-speed blender can handle tougher ingredients like nuts and seeds (if reintroduced).
5. **Instant Pot or Slow Cooker:** Great for making bone broth, stews, and tender meats without spending hours in the kitchen.
6. **Cast Iron Skillet:** Perfect for cooking meats and vegetables evenly. It's durable and adds a nice flavor to dishes.
7. **Baking Sheets and Parchment Paper:** Useful for roasting vegetables, baking AIP treats, and making crispy snacks.
8. **Glass Storage Containers:** Store leftovers and meal prepped foods in airtight glass containers to keep them fresh and easily accessible.
9. **Spiralizer:** Turn vegetables like zucchini and sweet potatoes into noodles for a fun, grain-free alternative to pasta.
10. **Immersion Blender:** Handy for pureeing soups and making sauces directly in the pot without transferring to a blender.

Ingredient Substitutions and Alternatives

When following the AIP diet, you might find that some of your favorite recipes need adjustments. Here are some common ingredient substitutions to help you adapt your recipes to be AIP-compliant:

1. **Grains and Flours:**
   - Replace Wheat Flour with coconut flour, cassava flour, or arrowroot powder.
   - Replace Rice with cauliflower rice or sweet potato rice.
2. **Dairy:**
   - Replace Milk with coconut milk or tigernut milk.
   - Replace Butter with coconut oil, avocado oil, or lard.
3. **Eggs:**
   - Replace Eggs in Baking with gelatin eggs (1 tablespoon gelatin + 2 tablespoons water) or mashed bananas/applesauce for binding.
4. **Legumes:**
   - Replace Beans in soups or stews with extra vegetables or shredded meat.
5. **Nightshades:**
   - Replace Tomatoes in sauces with a blend of beets, carrots, and pumpkin.
   - Replace Potatoes with sweet potatoes, turnips, or parsnips.
6. **Soy Sauce:**
   - Replace Soy Sauce with coconut aminos for a similar umami flavor.
7. **Sugar:**
   - Replace Refined Sugar with raw honey or maple syrup in moderation.

By stocking your pantry with AIP-friendly staples, equipping your kitchen with the right tools, and knowing how to make ingredient substitutions, you'll be well-prepared to cook delicious and compliant meals. Remember, the key to success on the AIP diet is preparation and creativity.

Meal Planning and Preparation Tips

Starting the AIP diet can seem overwhelming, but with a little planning and preparation, you can make the process smoother and more enjoyable. Let's look into some tips for weekly meal planning, grocery shopping, and batch cooking to help you stay on track and enjoy delicious, nourishing meals.

Weekly Meal Planning

Meal planning is a key strategy to ensure you always have AIP-friendly meals ready to go. Here's a step-by-step guide to help you plan your week:

1. **Set Aside Time for Planning:** Dedicate some time each week, like on a Sunday, to plan your meals. This helps you stay organized and reduces the stress of last-minute cooking.
2. **Create a Meal Calendar:** Use a simple calendar or planner to map out your meals for the week. Include breakfast, lunch, dinner, and snacks. This visual aid helps you see what you need to prepare.
3. **Balance Your Meals:** Ensure each meal includes a good balance of protein, healthy fats, and plenty of vegetables. For example, plan for a breakfast of scrambled eggs (if reintroduced) with sautéed spinach and avocado.
4. **Incorporate Variety:** Rotate different proteins and vegetables to keep your meals interesting and ensure you're getting a wide range of nutrients.
5. **Plan for Leftovers:** Cooking extra portions for dinner can provide easy lunches for the next day. This saves time and ensures you always have a meal ready.
6. **Include Treats:** Plan for AIP-friendly treats or snacks like fruit, homemade energy balls, or coconut yogurt with berries to satisfy cravings and keep you on track.

Grocery Shopping Tips

With your meal plan in hand, you're ready to tackle grocery shopping. Here are some tips to make your shopping trips efficient and AIP-compliant:

1. **Make a Detailed List:** Write down everything you need based on your meal plan. Organize your list by sections of the grocery store

(produce, meats, pantry items) to streamline your shopping.

2. **Shop the Perimeter:** Focus on the outer aisles of the store where fresh produce, meats, and fish are typically located. These areas usually have the least processed foods.

3. **Read Labels Carefully:** When buying packaged items, always check the ingredient list to ensure there are no hidden non-compliant ingredients like added sugars, preservatives, or nightshades.

4. **Buy in Bulk:**Purchase staples like coconut flour, olive oil, and canned coconut milk in bulk. This can save money and ensure you always have essential items on hand.

5. **Visit Local Farmers' Markets:** Farmers' markets are great places to find fresh, seasonal, and often organic produce. You can also ask vendors about their farming practices to ensure quality.

6. **Stock Up on Frozen Veggies:** Frozen vegetables are convenient and often just as nutritious as fresh ones. They're perfect for quick meals and can help reduce waste.

7. **Check for Sales and Deals:** Keep an eye out for sales on AIP staples and stock up when items are discounted. This can help you stay within your budget.

Batch Cooking and Meal Prep Strategies

Batch cooking and meal prepping are lifesavers when following the AIP diet. They save time and ensure you always have AIP-friendly meals ready. Here are some strategies to get you started:

1. **Cook in Batches:** Choose a few recipes each week that can be made in large quantities, like soups, stews, or casseroles. Cook these in batches and store them in the fridge or freezer for easy meals.

2. **Prep Ingredients Ahead of Time:** Spend some time washing, chopping, and portioning out vegetables and proteins. Store them in airtight containers so they're ready to use when you need them.

3. **Use Your Freezer:** Freeze portions of cooked meals for later use. Label containers with the date and contents so you can easily find what you need.

4. **Make Use of Kitchen Gadgets:** Use tools like slow cookers, Instant Pots, and food processors to save time. These gadgets can make cooking large batches easier and more efficient.

5. **Prepare Breakfasts in Advance:** Make breakfast items like chia pudding, overnight tigernut "oats," or egg muffins (if reintroduced) in advance. This ensures you have a nutritious start to your day.

6. **Plan for Snacks:** Prepare AIP-friendly snacks like vegetable sticks with guacamole, fruit, or homemade jerky. Having these on hand can help you avoid non-compliant foods when hunger strikes.

7. **Label and Organize:** Keep your fridge and pantry organized with labeled containers. This makes it easy to see what you have and prevents food from going to waste.

By incorporating these meal planning, grocery shopping, and meal prep strategies, you'll find it easier to stick to the AIP diet and enjoy a variety of delicious, nourishing meals. Remember, preparation is key to success, and a little effort up front can make a big difference in your AIP journey.

Chapter 2:

Breakfasts

1. Nutrient-Dense Breakfast Ideas

Starting your day with a nutrient-dense breakfast is essential for maintaining energy levels and keeping your immune system in check. Here are some AIP-friendly breakfast ideas that are not only delicious but also packed with nutrients. We've got you covered with smoothies, porridge alternatives, egg-free options, and AIP-compliant baked goodies.

Green Berry Smoothie

Nutritional Information (per serving):

- Calories: 200
- Protein: 3g
- Carbohydrates: 40g
- Fat: 6g
- Fiber: 8g

Ingredients:

- 1 cup spinach
- 1 cup mixed berries (blueberries, strawberries, raspberries)
- 1 banana
- 1 cup coconut milk
- 1 tablespoon coconut oil
- 1 tablespoon collagen peptides (optional, for added protein)

Instructions:

1. Place all ingredients in a blender.
2. Blend until smooth.
3. Pour into a glass and enjoy immediately.

Dietary Restriction Alternatives:

- For low-FODMAP: Replace banana with 1/2 cup of pineapple.
- For nut allergies: Ensure coconut milk is free from cross-contamination with nuts.

Tropical Smoothie Bowl

Nutritional Information (per serving):

- Calories: 350
- Protein: 5g
- Carbohydrates: 55g
- Fat: 15g
- Fiber: 10g

Ingredients:

- 1 cup mango chunks
- 1 cup pineapple chunks
- 1 banana
- 1 cup coconut milk
- 2 tablespoons coconut flakes
- 1 tablespoon pumpkin seeds (if tolerated)

Instructions:

1. Blend mango, pineapple, banana, and coconut milk until smooth.
2. Pour into a bowl.
3. Top with coconut flakes and pumpkin seeds.

Dietary Restriction Alternatives:

- **For low-FODMAP**: Replace banana with 1/2 cup of papaya.
- **For nut allergies**: Ensure pumpkin seeds are processed in a nut-free facility.

Grain-Free Porridge and Oatmeal Alternatives

Coconut and Apple Porridge

Nutritional Information (per serving):

- Calories: 250
- Protein: 4g
- Carbohydrates: 40g
- Fat: 12g
- Fiber: 6g

Ingredients:

- 1 cup unsweetened coconut flakes
- 1 apple, peeled and grated
- 1 cup coconut milk
- 1 tablespoon cinnamon
- 1 tablespoon maple syrup (optional)

Instructions:

1. In a pot, combine coconut flakes, grated apple, coconut milk, and cinnamon.
2. Cook over medium heat, stirring occasionally, until the mixture thickens (about 5-7 minutes).
3. Sweeten with maple syrup if desired.
4. Serve warm.

Dietary Alternatives:

- **For low-FODMAP**: Replace apple with 1/2 cup blueberries.
- **For nut allergies**: Ensure coconut flakes are processed in a nut-free facility.

Pumpkin Spice Porridge

Nutritional Information (per serving):

- Calories: 220
- Protein: 3g
- Carbohydrates: 30g
- Fat: 11g
- Fiber: 5g

Ingredients:

- 1 cup pumpkin puree
- 1/2 cup coconut milk
- 2 tablespoons tigernut flour
- 1 teaspoon cinnamon
- 1/2 teaspoon ground ginger
- 1/4 teaspoon nutmeg
- 1 tablespoon maple syrup (optional)

Instructions:

1. In a pot, combine pumpkin puree, coconut milk, tigernut flour, and spices.
2. Cook over medium heat, stirring frequently, until thickened (about 5 minutes).
3. Sweeten with maple syrup if desired.
4. Serve warm.

Dietary Alternatives:

- For low-FODMAP: Ensure portion size of pumpkin puree is appropriate.
- For nut allergies: Ensure tigernut flour is processed in a nut-free facility.

Egg-Free Breakfasts

Sweet Potato Hash

Nutritional Information (per serving):

- Calories: 180
- Protein: 2g
- Carbohydrates: 30g
- Fat: 7g
- Fiber: 4g

Ingredients:

- 2 medium sweet potatoes, peeled and diced
- 1 zucchini, diced
- 1 tablespoon coconut oil
- 1 teaspoon dried thyme
- Salt to taste

Instructions:

1. Heat coconut oil in a large skillet over medium heat.
2. Add diced sweet potatoes and cook for about 5 minutes, stirring occasionally.
3. Add zucchini and thyme, and cook for another 5 minutes, or until vegetables are tender.
4. Season with salt and serve warm.

Dietary Alternatives:

- **For low-FODMAP**: Replace zucchini with bell pepper (if tolerated).

Baked Apple with Cinnamon

Nutritional Information (per serving):

- Calories: 120
- Protein: 1g
- Carbohydrates: 29g
- Fat: 1g
- Fiber: 5g

Ingredients:

- 2 apples, cored and sliced
- 1 teaspoon cinnamon
- 1 tablespoon coconut oil
- 1 tablespoon honey (optional)

Instructions:

1. Preheat oven to 350°F (175°C).
2. Place apple slices in a baking dish.
3. Drizzle with coconut oil and sprinkle with cinnamon.
4. Bake for 20 minutes, or until apples are tender.
5. Drizzle with honey if desired and serve warm.

Dietary Alternatives:

- **For low-FODMAP**: Ensure portion size of apples is appropriate.
- For nut allergies: No changes needed.

Banana Tigernut Muffins

Nutritional Information (per muffin):

- Calories: 150
- Protein: 2g
- Carbohydrates: 25g
- Fat: 6g
- Fiber: 3g

Ingredients:

- 2 ripe bananas, mashed
- 1/2 cup tigernut flour
- 1/4 cup coconut flour
- 1/4 cup coconut oil, melted
- 1/2 teaspoon baking soda
- 1 teaspoon apple cider vinegar
- 1 teaspoon vanilla extract (optional)
- 1/4 teaspoon salt

Instructions:

1. Preheat oven to 350°F (175°C).
2. In a bowl, combine mashed bananas, coconut oil, and apple cider vinegar.
3. In another bowl, mix tigernut flour, coconut flour, baking soda, and salt.
4. Combine wet and dry ingredients, mixing until well blended.
5. Spoon batter into a muffin tin lined with paper liners.
6. Bake for 20-25 minutes, or until a toothpick inserted into the center comes out clean.
7. Let cool before serving.

Dietary Alternatives:

- **For low-FODMAP**: Replace bananas with a blend of 1/2 cup blueberries and 1/2 cup grated zucchini.

Coconut Flour Pancakes

Nutritional Information (per pancake):

- Calories: 90
- Protein: 2g
- Carbohydrates: 12g
- Fat: 4g
- Fiber: 3g

Ingredients:

- 1/2 cup coconut flour
- 1 cup coconut milk
- 1 tablespoon coconut oil, melted
- 1 teaspoon vanilla extract (optional)
- 1/4 teaspoon baking soda
- 1 tablespoon apple cider vinegar

Instructions:

1. In a bowl, mix coconut flour and baking soda.
2. Add coconut milk, coconut oil, vanilla extract, and apple cider vinegar. Stir until smooth.
3. Heat a skillet over medium heat and grease with a bit of coconut oil.
4. Pour 1/4 cup of batter onto the skillet and spread into a circle.
5. Cook for 2-3 minutes on each side, until golden brown.
6. Repeat with remaining batter.
7. Serve warm, optionally with a drizzle of honey or maple syrup.

Dietary Alternatives:

- **For low-FODMAP:** Ensure portion size of coconut flour is appropriate.

<h1 align="center">Sample Recipes</h1>

Sample Recipe 1: Herb-Roasted Chicken with Sweet Potato Mash

Nutritional Information (per serving):

- Calories: 350
- Protein: 25g
- Carbohydrates: 30g
- Fat: 15g
- Fiber: 5g

Ingredients:

- 4 bone-in, skin-on chicken thighs
- 2 sweet potatoes, peeled and cubed
- 2 tablespoons olive oil
- 1 tablespoon fresh rosemary, chopped
- 1 tablespoon fresh thyme, chopped
- Salt to taste
- 1 tablespoon coconut oil
- 1/4 cup coconut milk

Instructions:

1. Preheat oven to 400°F (200°C).
2. Place chicken thighs in a baking dish and drizzle with olive oil. Sprinkle with chopped rosemary, thyme, salt, and pepper.
3. Roast chicken in the preheated oven for 35-40 minutes, or until golden brown and cooked through.
4. While the chicken is roasting, boil sweet potatoes in a pot of water until tender, about 15-20 minutes.
5. Drain sweet potatoes and transfer them to a bowl. Add coconut oil and coconut milk. Mash until smooth and creamy. Season with salt to taste.
6. Serve roasted chicken thighs with sweet potato mash on the side.

- For low-FODMAP: Replace sweet potatoes with carrots or parsnips.
- For nut allergies: Use ghee instead of coconut oil.

Sample Recipe 2: Salmon and Asparagus Salad with Lemon Vinaigrette

Nutritional Information (per serving):

- Calories: 300
- Protein: 20g
- Carbohydrates: 15g
- Fat: 20g
- Fiber: 5g

Ingredients:

- 2 salmon fillets
- 1 bunch asparagus, trimmed
- 2 tablespoons olive oil
- Salt and pepper to taste
- 4 cups mixed greens
- 1/4 cup sliced almonds (optional)
- 1 lemon, juiced
- 2 tablespoons extra virgin olive oil
- 1 teaspoon honey (optional)
- 1 teaspoon Dijon mustard

Instructions:

1. Preheat oven to 400°F (200°C).
2. Place salmon fillets and asparagus on a baking sheet. Drizzle with olive oil and season with salt and pepper.
3. Roast in the preheated oven for 12-15 minutes, or until salmon is cooked through and asparagus is tender.

4. In a small bowl, whisk together lemon juice, extra virgin olive oil, honey (if using), and Dijon mustard to make the vinaigrette.
5. Divide mixed greens between plates. Top with roasted salmon and asparagus.
6. Drizzle with lemon vinaigrette and sprinkle with sliced almonds (if using).
7. Serve immediately.

Dietary Alternatives:

- For low-FODMAP: Omit honey from the vinaigrette.
- For nut allergies: Omit sliced almonds.

Sample Recipe 3: Beef and Vegetable Stir-Fry

Nutritional Information (per serving):

- Calories: 400
- Protein: 30g
- Carbohydrates: 25g
- Fat: 20g
- Fiber: 8g

Ingredients:

- 1 pound beef sirloin, thinly sliced
- 2 tablespoons coconut aminos
- 2 tablespoons olive oil
- 2 cups broccoli florets
- 1 red bell pepper, sliced
- 1 carrot, julienned
- 1 zucchini, sliced
- 2 cloves garlic, minced
- 1 tablespoon fresh ginger, minced
- Salt to taste

<u>Instructions</u>:

1. In a bowl, marinate beef slices in coconut aminos for 15-20 minutes.
2. Heat olive oil in a large skillet or wok over medium-high heat.
3. Add marinated beef slices and cook until browned, about 3-4 minutes. Remove from skillet and set aside.
4. In the same skillet, add broccoli, bell pepper, carrot, zucchini, garlic, and ginger. Stir-fry for 5-6 minutes, or until vegetables are tender-crisp.
5. Return cooked beef to the skillet and toss to combine with the vegetables.
6. Season with salt and pepper to taste.
7. Serve hot.

Dietary Alternatives:

- For low-FODMAP: Replace garlic with garlic-infused oil.
- For nut allergies: No changes needed.

Chapter 3:

Snacks and Appetizers

1. Healthy Snack Options

When following the AIP diet, having convenient and satisfying snacks on hand can help you stay on track and avoid temptation. Here are some delicious and nutrient-packed snack ideas that are perfect for any occasion.

Portable Snacks

<u>Nut and Seed Trail Mix</u>

<u>Nutritional Information (per serving):</u>

- Calories: 200
- Protein: 5g
- Carbohydrates: 15g
- Fat: 14g
- Fiber: 4g

<u>Ingredients:</u>

- 1/2 cup mixed nuts (almonds, cashews, walnuts)
- 1/4 cup pumpkin seeds
- 1/4 cup dried fruit (raisins, cranberries, apricots)
- 2 tablespoons coconut flakes

<u>Instructions:</u>

1. Mix all ingredients together in a bowl.
2. Divide into individual portions in resealable bags for easy grab-and-go snacks.

<u>Dietary Alternatives:</u>

- For nut allergies: Replace nuts with roasted chickpeas or additional seeds.

Apple Slices with Almond Butter

Nutritional Information (per serving):

- Calories: 150
- Protein: 3g
- Carbohydrates: 20g
- Fat: 7g
- Fiber: 5g

Ingredients:

- 1 apple, sliced
- 2 tablespoons almond butter

Instructions:

1. Spread almond butter on apple slices.
2. Enjoy immediately.

Dietary Alternatives:

- For nut allergies: Replace almond butter with sunflower seed butter or coconut butter.

<u>Guacamole with Veggie Sticks</u>

<u>Nutritional Information (per serving):</u>

- Calories: 150
- Protein: 3g
- Carbohydrates: 10g
- Fat: 12g
- Fiber: 7g

<u>Ingredients:</u>

- 2 ripe avocados
- 1 tomato, diced
- 1/4 cup chopped cilantro
- 1/4 cup diced red onion (optional, omit if sensitive)
- Juice of 1 lime
- Salt and pepper to taste
- Carrot and cucumber sticks for dipping

<u>Instructions:</u>

1. Scoop avocado flesh into a bowl and mash with a fork.
2. Stir in diced tomato, chopped cilantro, diced red onion (if using), lime juice, salt, and pepper.
3. Serve with carrot and cucumber sticks for dipping.

<u>Dietary Alternatives:</u>

- For low-FODMAP: Omit red onion.
- For avocado allergies: Replace guacamole with mashed cooked sweet potato mixed with lime juice and salt.

<u>Tahini Dip with Crudites</u>

<u>Nutritional Information (per serving):</u>

- Calories: 120
- Protein: 4g
- Carbohydrates: 8g
- Fat: 8g
- Fiber: 4g

<u>Ingredients</u>:

- 1/4 cup tahini
- 2 tablespoons lemon juice
- 1 clove garlic, minced (optional, omit if sensitive)
- 1/4 teaspoon ground cumin
- Salt to taste
- Assorted vegetable sticks (carrots, celery, cucumber)

<u>Instructions:</u>

1. In a bowl, whisk together tahini, lemon juice, minced garlic (if using), ground cumin, and salt until smooth.
2. Adjust seasoning to taste.
3. Serve with assorted vegetable sticks for dipping.

<u>*Dietary Alternatives:*</u>

- For low-FODMAP: Omit garlic.
- For sesame seed allergies: Replace tahini with sunflower seed butter.

Crispy Sweet Potato Chips

Nutritional Information (per serving):

- Calories: 120
- Protein: 2g
- Carbohydrates: 20g
- Fat: 4g
- Fiber: 3g

Ingredients:

- 2 medium sweet potatoes, peeled and thinly sliced
- 2 tablespoons olive oil
- Salt to taste

Instructions:

1. Preheat oven to 375°F (190°C).
2. Toss sweet potato slices with olive oil and salt in a bowl until evenly coated.
3. Arrange sweet potato slices in a single layer on a baking sheet.
4. Bake for 15-20 minutes, or until crispy and golden brown.
5. Let cool before serving.

Dietary Alternatives:

- For low-FODMAP: Ensure portion size of sweet potatoes is appropriate.
- For nightshade allergies: Replace sweet potatoes with carrots or parsnips.

Cucumber and Radish Roll-Ups

Nutritional Information (per serving):

- Calories: 40
- Protein: 1g
- Carbohydrates: 5g
- Fat: 2g
- Fiber: 2g

Ingredients:

- 1 large cucumber
- 4-6 radishes
- 1/4 cup guacamole or hummus (optional)

Instructions:

1. Use a mandoline or vegetable peeler to slice the cucumber lengthwise into thin strips.
2. Thinly slice the radishes.
3. Place a spoonful of guacamole or hummus (if using) at one end of each cucumber strip.
4. Add a few slices of radish on top of the guacamole or hummus.
5. Roll up the cucumber strip tightly, enclosing the filling.
6. Secure with a toothpick if needed.
7. Repeat with remaining cucumber strips and radish slices.
8. Serve immediately or refrigerate until ready to eat.

Dietary Alternatives:

- For low-FODMAP: Omit guacamole or hummus and use plain cucumber slices rolled with radish slices.
- For cucumber allergies: Replace cucumber with zucchini slices.

Sample recipes

Recipe 1: Herb-Crusted Salmon with Roasted Vegetables

Nutritional Information (per serving):

- Calories: 300
- Protein: 25g
- Carbohydrates: 20g
- Fat: 15g
- Fiber: 5g

Ingredients:

- 2 salmon fillets
- 1 tablespoon olive oil
- 1 tablespoon fresh parsley, chopped
- 1 tablespoon fresh dill, chopped
- 1 teaspoon garlic powder
- Salt to taste
- 2 cups mixed vegetables (e.g., carrots, broccoli, cauliflower), chopped
- 1 tablespoon coconut oil, melted

Instructions:

1. Preheat oven to 400°F (200°C).
2. Place salmon fillets on a baking sheet lined with parchment paper.
3. In a small bowl, mix together olive oil, parsley, dill, garlic powder, salt, and pepper.
4. Brush the herb mixture evenly over the salmon fillets.
5. In another bowl, toss mixed vegetables with melted coconut oil and salt.
6. Arrange vegetables around the salmon on the baking sheet.

7. Roast in the preheated oven for 15-20 minutes, or until salmon is cooked through and vegetables are tender.
8. Serve hot.

Dietary Alternatives:

- For low-FODMAP: Use carrots, zucchini, and green beans as vegetables.
- For fish allergies: Replace salmon with chicken breast or tofu.

Recipe 2: Beef and Mushroom Stir-Fry

Nutritional Information (per serving):

- Calories: 350
- Protein: 30g
- Carbohydrates: 15g
- Fat: 20g
- Fiber: 4g

Ingredients:

- 1 pound beef sirloin, thinly sliced
- 2 tablespoons coconut aminos
- 1 tablespoon coconut oil
- 2 cups mixed mushrooms, sliced
- 1 cup broccoli florets
- 2 cloves garlic, minced
- 1 tablespoon fresh ginger, minced
- Salt to taste
- 2 green onions, sliced (optional)

Instructions:

1. In a bowl, marinate beef slices in coconut aminos for 15-20 minutes.
2. Heat coconut oil in a large skillet or wok over medium-high heat.

3. Add marinated beef slices and cook until browned, about 3-4 minutes. Remove from skillet and set aside.
4. In the same skillet, add mushrooms and cook until they release their liquid and start to brown, about 5 minutes.
5. Add broccoli florets, minced garlic, and minced ginger to the skillet. Cook for another 3-4 minutes, or until broccoli is tender-crisp.
6. Return cooked beef to the skillet and toss to combine with the vegetables.
7. Season with salt to taste.
8. Garnish with sliced green onions (if using) and serve hot.

Dietary Alternatives:

- For low-FODMAP: Omit garlic and use only green parts of green onions.
- For mushroom allergies: Replace mushrooms with bell peppers or snap peas.

Recipe 3: Baked Chicken Drumsticks with Sweet Potato Fries

Nutritional Information (per serving):

- Calories: 400
- Protein: 25g
- Carbohydrates: 30g
- Fat: 20g
- Fiber: 5g

Ingredients:

- 4 chicken drumsticks
- 2 tablespoons olive oil
- 1 tablespoon fresh thyme, chopped
- 1 tablespoon fresh rosemary, chopped
- Salt and pepper to taste
- 2 medium sweet potatoes, cut into fries
- 1 tablespoon coconut oil, melted

<h1 style="text-align:center"><u>Instructions:</u></h1>

1. Preheat oven to 400°F (200°C).
2. Place chicken drumsticks on a baking sheet lined with parchment paper.
3. In a small bowl, mix together olive oil, thyme, rosemary and salt.
4. Brush the herb mixture evenly over the chicken drumsticks.
5. In another bowl, toss sweet potato fries with melted coconut oil, salt, and pepper.
6. Arrange sweet potato fries around the chicken drumsticks on the baking sheet.
7. Bake in the preheated oven for 35-40 minutes, or until chicken is cooked through and sweet potato fries are crispy.
8. Serve hot.

<u>Dietary Alternatives:</u>

- For low-FODMAP: Ensure portion size of sweet potatoes is appropriate.
- For poultry allergies: Replace chicken drumsticks with turkey drumsticks or pork chops.

Chapter 4:

Soups and Salads

1. Healing Soups and Stews

Warm, comforting, and nourishing, soups and stews are perfect for soothing the body and providing essential nutrients. Here are some healing recipes that are gentle on the digestive system and packed with flavor.

Bone Broths

Nutritional Information (per serving):

- Calories: 50
- Protein: 10g
- Carbohydrates: 0g
- Fat: 1g
- Fiber: 0g

Ingredients:

- 2-3 pounds beef or chicken bones
- 2 carrots, chopped
- 2 celery stalks, chopped
- 1 onion, quartered (if tolerated)
- 2 garlic cloves, smashed
- 1 tablespoon apple cider vinegar
- Salt to taste
- Water

Instructions:

1. Preheat oven to 400°F (200°C).
2. Place bones, carrots, celery, onion, (if using) and garlic on a baking sheet. Roast for 30 minutes.
3. Transfer roasted bones and vegetables to a large stockpot. Add apple cider vinegar and enough water to cover the ingredients.

4. Bring to a boil, then reduce heat to low and simmer, covered, for 8-24 hours.
5. Skim off any foam that rises to the surface.
6. Strain the broth through a fine-mesh sieve or cheesecloth.
7. Season with salt and pepper to taste.
8. Store in the refrigerator for up to 5 days or freeze for later use.

Dietary Alternatives:

- For low-FODMAP: Omit onion and garlic.
- For vegetarians: Use vegetable scraps and omit bones.

Vegetable Soups

Nutritional Information (per serving):

- Calories: 150
- Protein: 4g
- Carbohydrates: 20g
- Fat: 6g
- Fiber: 5g

Ingredients:

- 1 tablespoon coconut oil
- 2 carrots, chopped
- 2 celery stalks, chopped
- 2 cups chopped seasonal vegetables (e.g., broccoli, cauliflower, zucchini)
- 4 cups bone broth or vegetable broth
- 1 teaspoon dried thyme
- Salt to taste
- Fresh herbs for garnish (optional)

Instructions:

1. Heat coconut oil in a large pot over medium heat.
2. Add carrots, and celery. Cook until softened, about 5 minutes.
3. Add seasonal vegetables and cook for another 3-4 minutes.
4. Pour in bone broth or vegetable broth. Add dried thyme and salt
5. Bring to a boil, then reduce heat to low and simmer, covered, for 20-25 minutes, or until vegetables are tender.
6. Use an immersion blender to blend the soup until smooth. Alternatively, transfer soup to a blender and blend in batches until smooth.
7. Adjust seasoning if needed.
8. Serve hot, garnished with fresh herbs if desired.

Dietary Alternatives:

- For low-FODMAP: Use low-FODMAP vegetables such as carrots, zucchini, and green beans.
- For nightshade allergies: Avoid tomatoes and peppers.

Meat-Based Stews

Nutritional Information (per serving):

- Calories: 300
- Protein: 25g
- Carbohydrates: 15g
- Fat: 15g
- Fiber: 3g

Ingredients:

- 1 pound stewing beef, cubed
- 2 tablespoons coconut oi
- 2 carrots, chopped
- 2 celery stalks, chopped
- 2 cups chopped potatoes (or sweet potatoes for AIP)
- 4 cups bone broth
- 1 teaspoon dried thyme

- Salt and little pepper to taste
- Fresh parsley for garnish (optional)

Instructions:

1. Heat coconut oil in a large pot over medium heat.
2. Add cubed beef and cook until browned on all sides, about 5 minutes.
3. Add carrots, and celery. Cook until softened, about 5 minutes.
4. Stir in chopped potatoes, bone broth, dried thyme, salt, and pepper.
5. Bring to a boil, then reduce heat to low and simmer, covered, for 1-2 hours, or until beef is tender.
6. Adjust seasoning if needed.
7. Serve hot, garnished with fresh parsley if desired.

Dietary Alternatives:

- For low-FODMAP: Use low-FODMAP vegetables such as carrots and green beans.
- For nightshade allergies: Omit tomatoes and peppers.

<u>Refreshing Salads</u>

Salads are not only nutritious but also versatile and refreshing. Whether you're looking for a light meal or a flavorful side dish, these salad recipes are sure to delight your taste buds while providing essential nutrients.

Salad Dressings and Vinaigrettes
<u>Basic Balsamic Vinaigrette</u>

<u>Nutritional Information (per serving):</u>

- Calories: 60
- Protein: 0g
- Carbohydrates: 3g
- Fat: 6g
- Fiber: 0g

<u>Ingredients:</u>

- 3 tablespoons extra virgin olive oil
- 1 tablespoon balsamic vinegar
- 1 teaspoon Dijon mustard
- Salt to taste

<u>Instructions:</u>

1. In a small bowl, whisk together olive oil, balsamic vinegar, and Dijon mustard until well combined.
2. Season with salt to taste.
3. Drizzle over your favorite salad and toss to coat.

<u>Dietary Alternatives:</u>

- For low-FODMAP: Use maple syrup instead of balsamic vinegar.
- For mustard allergies: Omit Dijon mustard or use a pinch of dried herbs for flavor.

Protein-Packed Salads
<u>Grilled Chicken and Avocado Salad</u>

<u>Nutritional Information (per serving):</u>

- Calories: 300
- Protein: 25g
- Carbohydrates: 10g
- Fat: 15g
- Fiber: 5g

<u>Ingredients:</u>

- 2 boneless, skinless chicken breasts
- 1 tablespoon olive oil
- Salt to taste
- 4 cups mixed greens
- 1 avocado, diced
- 1/4 cup sliced almonds
- Balsamic vinaigrette (see recipe above)

<u>Instructions:</u>

1. Preheat grill or grill pan over medium-high heat.
2. Brush chicken breasts with olive oil and season with salt and pepper.
3. Grill chicken for 6-8 minutes per side, or until cooked through and no longer pink in the center.
4. Let chicken rest for a few minutes, then slice into strips.
5. In a large bowl, combine mixed greens, diced avocado, sliced almonds, and grilled chicken strips.
6. Drizzle with balsamic vinaigrette and toss to coat.
7. Serve immediately.

<u>Dietary Alternatives:</u>

- For nut allergies: Omit sliced almonds or replace with sunflower seeds.
- For avocado allergies: Replace avocado with sliced cucumber or diced bell peppers.

Summer Berry Spinach Salad

Nutritional Information (per serving):

- Calories: 200
- Protein: 5g
- Carbohydrates: 20g
- Fat: 10g
- Fiber: 8g

Ingredients:

- 4 cups fresh spinach leaves
- 1 cup mixed berries (strawberries, blueberries, raspberries)
- 1/4 cup sliced almonds
- 2 tablespoons crumbled goat cheese (optional)
- Lemon vinaigrette (see recipe below)

Instructions:

1. In a large bowl, combine fresh spinach leaves, mixed berries, sliced almonds, and crumbled goat cheese (if using).
2. Drizzle with lemon vinaigrette and toss gently to coat.
3. Serve immediately.

Dietary Alternatives:

- For nut allergies: Omit sliced almonds.
- For dairy allergies: Omit crumbled goat cheese or replace with dairy-free cheese alternative.

Lemon Vinaigrette

Nutritional Information (per serving):

- Calories: 50
- Protein: 0g
- Carbohydrates: 3g
- Fat: 5g
- Fiber: 0g

Ingredients:

- 3 tablespoons extra virgin olive oil
- 2 tablespoons fresh lemon juice
- 1 teaspoon honey (optional)
- Salt to taste

Instructions:

1. In a small bowl, whisk together olive oil, lemon juice, and honey (if using) until well combined.
2. Season with salt to taste.
3. Drizzle over your favorite salad and toss to coat.

Dietary Alternatives:

- For low-FODMAP: Omit honey.
- For citrus allergies: Replace lemon juice with apple cider vinegar.

More Soup Recipes

Recipe 1: Butternut Squash Soup

Nutritional Information (per serving):

- Calories: 150
- Protein: 2g
- Carbohydrates: 30g
- Fat: 3g
- Fiber: 5g

Ingredients:

- 1 medium butternut squash, peeled, seeded, and diced
- 1 tablespoon coconut oil
- 1 apple, peeled, cored, and diced
- 1 teaspoon ground cinnamon
- 1/2 teaspoon ground nutmeg
- 4 cups vegetable broth
- Salt to taste
- Coconut cream for garnish (optional)

Instructions:

1. Heat coconut oil in a large pot over medium heat.
2. Add diced butternut squash and apple to the pot. Cook until slightly softened, about 5 minutes.
3. Stir in ground cinnamon and ground nutmeg.
4. Pour in vegetable broth and bring to a boil.
5. Reduce heat to low, cover, and simmer for 20-25 minutes, or until squash is tender.
6. Use an immersion blender to puree the soup until smooth. Alternatively, transfer the soup to a blender and blend until smooth.
7. Season with salt to taste.
8. Serve hot, garnished with a dollop of coconut cream if desired.

Recipe 2: Chicken and Vegetable Soup

Nutritional Information (per serving):

- Calories: 200
- Protein: 20g
- Carbohydrates: 15g
- Fat: 6g
- Fiber: 4g

Ingredients:

- 1 tablespoon olive oil
- 2 boneless, skinless chicken breasts, diced
- 2 carrots, peeled and sliced
- 2 celery stalks, sliced
- 1 cup chopped kale
- 4 cups chicken broth
- 1 teaspoon dried thyme
- Salt to taste
- Fresh parsley for garnish (optional)

Instructions:

1. Heat olive oil in a large pot over medium heat.
2. Add diced chicken breasts to the pot. Cook until browned on all sides, about 5 minutes.
3. Add sliced carrots and celery to the pot. Cook for another 3-4 minutes.
4. Stir in chopped kale, chicken broth, and dried thyme.
5. Bring to a boil, then reduce heat to low and simmer, covered, for 20-25 minutes, or until vegetables are tender and chicken is cooked through.
6. Season with salt to taste.
7. Serve hot, garnished with fresh parsley if desired.

Recipe 3: Lentil Soup

Nutritional Information (per serving):

- Calories: 250
- Protein: 15g
- Carbohydrates: 40g
- Fat: 2g
- Fiber: 15g

Ingredients:

- 1 cup dried green lentils, rinsed and drained
- 1 tablespoon olive oil
- 1 carrot, peeled and diced
- 1 celery stalk, diced
- 1 small sweet potato, peeled and diced
- 1 teaspoon ground cumin
- 1/2 teaspoon ground turmeric
- 4 cups vegetable broth
- Salt to taste
- Fresh cilantro for garnish (optional)

Instructions:

1. In a large pot, heat olive oil over medium heat.
2. Add diced carrot, celery, and sweet potato to the pot. Cook until slightly softened, about 5 minutes.
3. Stir in ground cumin and ground turmeric.
4. Add rinsed lentils and vegetable broth to the pot. Bring to a boil.
5. Reduce heat to low, cover, and simmer for 20-25 minutes, or until lentils and vegetables are tender.
6. Season with salt and pepper to taste.
7. Serve hot, garnished with fresh cilantro if desired.

Dietary Alternatives:

- For low-FODMAP: Use canned lentils instead of dried lentils.
- For legume allergies: Replace lentils with quinoa or rice.

Chapter 5:

Main Dishes

Herb-Roasted Chicken

Nutritional Information (per serving):

- Calories: 300
- Protein: 25g
- Carbohydrates: 0g
- Fat: 20g
- Fiber: 0g

Ingredients:

- 4 bone-in, skin-on chicken thighs
- 2 tablespoons olive oil
- 1 tablespoon fresh rosemary, chopped
- 1 tablespoon fresh thyme, chopped
- Salt to taste

Instructions:

1. Preheat oven to 400°F (200°C).
2. Rub chicken thighs with olive oil and season with chopped rosemary, thyme and salt,.
3. Place chicken thighs on a baking sheet lined with parchment paper.
4. Roast in the preheated oven for 35-40 minutes, or until chicken is golden brown and cooked through.
5. Serve hot.

Dietary Alternatives:

- For low-FODMAP: Omit garlic and onion from the herb mixture.
- For poultry allergies: Replace chicken thighs with bone-in, skin-on turkey thighs.

Braised Beef Short Ribs

Nutritional Information (per serving):

- Calories: 400
- Protein: 30g
- Carbohydrates: 10g
- Fat: 25g
- Fiber: 2g

Ingredients:

- 4 beef short ribs
- 2 tablespoons coconut oil
- 1 onion, chopped
- 2 carrots, chopped
- 2 celery stalks, chopped
- 2 cloves garlic, minced
- 2 cups beef broth
- 1 cup red wine (optional)
- Salt to taste

Instructions:

1. Preheat oven to 325°F (160°C).
2. Season beef short ribs with salt.
3. Heat coconut oil in a Dutch oven over medium-high heat.
4. Sear beef short ribs until browned on all sides, about 5 minutes per side. Remove from the pot and set aside.
5. In the same pot, add chopped onion, carrots, celery, and minced garlic. Cook until softened, about 5 minutes.
6. Return beef short ribs to the pot. Add beef broth and red wine (if using).
7. Bring to a boil, then cover and transfer to the preheated oven.
8. Braise in the oven for 2-3 hours, or until beef is tender and falling off the bone.
9. Serve hot, spooning the sauce over the beef short ribs.

Dietary Alternatives:

- For low-FODMAP: Omit onion and garlic.
- For alcohol-free: Replace red wine with additional beef broth.

Baked Lemon Herb Salmon

Nutritional Information (per serving):

- Calories: 250
- Protein: 25g
- Carbohydrates: 2g
- Fat: 15g
- Fiber: 1g

Ingredients:

- 2 salmon fillets
- 2 tablespoons olive oil
- 1 lemon, thinly sliced
- 2 cloves garlic, minced
- 1 teaspoon dried dill
- Salt to taste
- Fresh parsley for garnish (optional)

Instructions:

1. Preheat oven to 375°F (190°C).
2. Place salmon fillets on a baking sheet lined with parchment paper.
3. Drizzle olive oil over the salmon fillets.
4. Top with lemon slices and minced garlic.
5. Sprinkle dried dill and salt over the salmon.
6. Bake in the preheated oven for 12-15 minutes, or until salmon is cooked through and flakes easily with a fork.
7. Garnish with fresh parsley before serving.

Dietary Alternatives:

- For low-FODMAP: Omit garlic.
- For vegetarian: Substitute salmon with firm tofu and adjust baking time as needed.

Garlic Butter Shrimp

Nutritional Information (per serving):

- Calories: 200
- Protein: 20g
- Carbohydrates: 2g
- Fat: 12g
- Fiber: 0g

Ingredients:

- 1 pound large shrimp, peeled and deveined
- 2 tablespoons unsalted butter
- 3 cloves garlic, minced
- 1 tablespoon fresh parsley, chopped
- Salt to taste
- Lemon wedges for serving (optional)

Instructions:

1. Heat butter in a large skillet over medium heat.
2. Add minced garlic to the skillet and cook until fragrant, about 1 minute.
3. Add shrimp to the skillet and cook until pink and opaque, about 2-3 minutes per side.
4. Season with salt and chopped parsley.
5. Serve hot with lemon wedges on the side.

Dietary Alternatives:

- For low-FODMAP: Omit garlic and use garlic-infused oil.
- For dairy-free: Replace butter with olive oil.

Vegetarian Main Dishes

Portobello Mushroom Steaks

Nutritional Information (per serving):

- Calories: 150
- Protein: 5g
- Carbohydrates: 10g
- Fat: 10g
- Fiber: 4g

Ingredients:

- 4 large portobello mushroom caps
- 2 tablespoons balsamic vinegar
- 2 tablespoons olive oil
- 2 cloves garlic, minced
- 1 teaspoon dried thyme
- Salt to taste
- Fresh parsley for garnish (optional)

Instructions:

1. Clean the portobello mushroom caps and remove the stems.
2. In a shallow dish, whisk together balsamic vinegar, olive oil, minced garlic, dried thyme, salt, and pepper.
3. Place mushroom caps in the marinade, turning to coat evenly. Let marinate for at least 30 minutes.
4. Preheat grill or grill pan over medium-high heat.
5. Grill mushroom caps for 4-5 minutes per side, or until tender and grill marks appear.
6. Serve hot, garnished with fresh parsley if desired.

Dietary Alternatives:

- For low-FODMAP: Omit garlic.

- For vegan: Replace balsamic vinegar with tamari or soy sauce and ensure other ingredients are vegan-friendly.

Lentil and Vegetable Stir-Fry

Nutritional Information (per serving):

- Calories: 250
- Protein: 12g
- Carbohydrates: 40g
- Fat: 5g
- Fiber: 10g

Ingredients:

- 1 cup dried green lentils, cooked
- 2 tablespoons sesame oil
- 2 cups mixed vegetables (bell peppers, broccoli, carrots, snap peas)
- 2 cloves garlic, minced
- 1 tablespoon fresh ginger, minced
- 2 tablespoons soy sauce or tamari
- 1 tablespoon rice vinegar
- 1 teaspoon honey (optional)
- Sesame seeds for garnish (optional)

Instructions:

1. Heat sesame oil in a large skillet or wok over medium-high heat.
2. Add minced garlic and ginger to the skillet. Cook until fragrant, about 1 minute.
3. Add mixed vegetables to the skillet and stir-fry until crisp-tender, about 5-6 minutes.
4. Stir in cooked lentils.
5. In a small bowl, whisk together soy sauce or tamari, rice vinegar, and honey (if using). Pour over the vegetable and lentil mixture.

6. Cook for another 2-3 minutes, stirring constantly, until everything is heated through and coated in the sauce.
7. Garnish with sesame seeds before serving.

Dietary Alternatives:

- For low-FODMAP: Use low-FODMAP vegetables such as carrots and bell peppers.
- For gluten-free: Ensure soy sauce or tamari is gluten-free.

More Main Dishes Recipes

Recipe 1: Vegetable Stir-Fry with Tofu

Nutritional Information (per serving):

- Calories: 250
- Protein: 15g
- Carbohydrates: 20g
- Fat: 12g
- Fiber: 6g

Ingredients:

- 1 block firm tofu, pressed and cubed
- 2 tablespoons sesame oil
- 2 cups mixed vegetables (bell peppers, broccoli, carrots, snap peas)
- 2 cloves garlic, minced
- 1 tablespoon fresh ginger, minced
- 2 tablespoons soy sauce or tamari
- 1 tablespoon rice vinegar
- 1 teaspoon honey or maple syrup (optional)
- Sesame seeds for garnish (optional)
- Cooked rice or quinoa for serving

Instructions:

1. Heat sesame oil in a large skillet or wok over medium-high heat.
2. Add cubed tofu to the skillet and cook until golden brown on all sides, about 5-7 minutes. Remove tofu from the skillet and set aside.
3. In the same skillet, add minced garlic and ginger. Cook until fragrant, about 1 minute.
4. Add mixed vegetables to the skillet and stir-fry until crisp-tender, about 5-6 minutes.
5. Return cooked tofu to the skillet.
6. In a small bowl, whisk together soy sauce or tamari, rice vinegar, and honey or maple syrup (if using). Pour over the tofu and vegetable mixture.
7. Cook for another 2-3 minutes, stirring constantly, until everything is heated through and coated in the sauce.
8. Garnish with sesame seeds before serving.
9. Serve hot with cooked rice or quinoa.

Dietary Alternatives:

- For low-FODMAP: Use low-FODMAP vegetables such as carrots and bell peppers.
- For gluten-free: Ensure soy sauce or tamari is gluten-free.

Recipe 2: Spaghetti Squash with Tomato Basil Sauce

Nutritional Information (per serving):

- Calories: 200
- Protein: 4g
- Carbohydrates: 30g
- Fat: 8g
- Fiber: 6g

Ingredients:

- 1 spaghetti squash
- 2 tablespoons olive oil
- 2 cloves garlic, minced
- 1 can (14 oz) diced tomatoes
- 1/4 cup fresh basil, chopped
- Salt to taste
- Vegan parmesan cheese for garnish (optional)

Instructions:

1. Preheat oven to 400°F (200°C).
2. Cut spaghetti squash in half lengthwise and remove the seeds.
3. Drizzle olive oil over the cut sides of the spaghetti squash and season with salt and pepper.
4. Place squash halves, cut side down, on a baking sheet lined with parchment paper.
5. Roast in the preheated oven for 40-45 minutes, or until squash is tender and easily pierced with a fork.
6. While the squash is roasting, heat olive oil in a skillet over medium heat.
7. Add minced garlic to the skillet and cook until fragrant, about 1 minute.
8. Stir in diced tomatoes and chopped basil. Cook for another 5-7 minutes, or until heated through.
9. Use a fork to scrape the flesh of the spaghetti squash into strands.
10. Divide the spaghetti squash strands among plates and top with tomato basil sauce.
11. Garnish with vegan parmesan cheese before serving, if desired.

Dietary Alternatives:

- For low-FODMAP: Omit garlic.
- For vegan: Use vegan parmesan cheese or nutritional yeast for garnish.

<h1 style="text-align:center"><u>Recipe 3: Cauliflower and Chickpea Curry</u></h1>

<u>Nutritional Information (per serving):</u>

- Calories: 300
- Protein: 10g
- Carbohydrates: 40g
- Fat: 12g
- Fiber: 10g

<u>Ingredients:</u>

- 1 head cauliflower, cut into florets
- 1 can (14 oz) chickpeas, drained and rinsed
- 1 tablespoon coconut oil
- 1 onion, chopped
- 2 cloves garlic, minced
- 1 tablespoon fresh ginger, minced
- 2 tablespoons curry powder
- 1 can (14 oz) coconut milk
- 1 cup vegetable broth
- Salt and pepper to taste
- Fresh cilantro for garnish (optional)
- Cooked rice or naan bread for serving

Instructions:

1. Heat coconut oil in a large skillet or pot over medium heat.
2. Add chopped onion, minced garlic, and minced ginger. Cook until onion is translucent, about 5 minutes.
3. Stir in curry powder and cook for another 1-2 minutes, until fragrant.
4. Add cauliflower florets and chickpeas to the skillet. Stir to coat in the curry mixture.
5. Pour in coconut milk and vegetable broth. Bring to a simmer.
6. Cover and cook for 15-20 minutes, or until cauliflower is tender.
7. 7. Season with salt and pepper to taste.
8. Serve hot, garnished with fresh cilantro if desired.

9. Serve over cooked rice or with naan bread on the side.

Dietary Alternatives:

- For low-FODMAP: Omit garlic and onion.
- For gluten-free: Serve with gluten-free naan bread or over cooked quinoa instead of rice.

Chapter 6:

AIP-friendly Side Dishes

Complementary Sides

In this chapter, we explore a variety of AIP-friendly side dishes that perfectly complement your main courses. From nutrient-packed vegetables and greens to satisfying grain-free starches and the benefits of fermented foods, these side dishes will elevate your meals without compromising your dietary restrictions.

Roasted Garlic Herb Carrots

Nutritional Information (per serving):

- Calories: 100
- Protein: 2g
- Carbohydrates: 15g
- Fat: 5g
- Fiber: 4g

Ingredients:

- 1 pound carrots, peeled and sliced into sticks
- 2 tablespoons olive oil
- 2 cloves garlic, minced
- 1 teaspoon dried thyme
- Salt to taste
- Fresh parsley for garnish (optional)

Instructions:

1. Preheat oven to 400°F (200°C).
2. In a large bowl, toss carrot sticks with olive oil, minced garlic, dried thyme, salt, until evenly coated.
3. Spread carrots in a single layer on a baking sheet lined with parchment paper.
4. Roast in the preheated oven for 20-25 minutes, or until carrots are tender and lightly browned, stirring halfway through.
5. Garnish with fresh parsley before serving.

Dietary Alternatives:

- For low-FODMAP: Omit garlic.
- For nightshade-free: Substitute carrots with parsnips or sweet potatoes.

Garlic Mashed Cauliflower

Nutritional Information (per serving):

- Calories: 80
- Protein: 3g
- Carbohydrates: 10g
- Fat: 4g
- Fiber: 4g

Ingredients:

- 1 head cauliflower, cut into florets
- 2 tablespoons coconut cream
- 2 cloves garlic, minced
- 1 tablespoon olive oil
- Salt to taste
- Chopped chives for garnish (optional)

Instructions:

1. Steam cauliflower florets until tender, about 10-12 minutes.
2. Transfer steamed cauliflower to a food processor.
3. Add coconut cream, minced garlic, olive oil and salt to the food processor.
4. Blend until smooth and creamy, scraping down the sides as needed.
5. Taste and adjust seasoning if necessary.
6. Transfer mashed cauliflower to a serving dish and garnish with chopped chives if desired.

Dietary Alternatives:

- For low-FODMAP: Omit garlic.
- For nut-free: Substitute coconut cream with full-fat coconut milk.

Fermented Foods and Their Benefits

Homemade Sauerkraut

Nutritional Information (per serving):

- Calories: 15
- Protein: 1g
- Carbohydrates: 3g
- Fat: 0g
- Fiber: 2g

Ingredients:

- 1 head green cabbage, shredded
- 1 tablespoon sea salt
- Caraway seeds (optional)

Instructions:

1. In a large bowl, combine shredded cabbage and sea salt.
2. Massage the cabbage with your hands for 5-10 minutes, or until it starts to release liquid.
3. Pack the cabbage tightly into a clean glass jar, pressing down to submerge it in its own juices.
4. Add caraway seeds on top if desired.
5. Cover the jar with a clean cloth or lid, but do not seal it completely.
6. Let the jar sit at room temperature for 1-2 weeks, checking every few days to ensure the cabbage remains submerged.
7. Once fermented to your liking, seal the jar and store it in the refrigerator.
8. Serve sauerkraut as a tangy and probiotic-rich side dish to complement your meals.

Dietary Alternatives:

- For low-sodium: Use less salt in the fermentation process.
- For cabbage allergies: Substitute cabbage with shredded carrots or radishes.

BENEFITS OF FERMENTED FOODS

Fermented foods offer a variety of health benefits, particularly for gut health and overall well-being. Here are some key benefits of including fermented foods in your diet:

1. Improved Digestive Health

Probiotics:
Fermented foods are rich in probiotics, which are beneficial bacteria that support a healthy gut microbiome. These probiotics can help balance the gut flora, promoting better digestion and nutrient absorption.

Enhanced Digestion:
Fermentation breaks down complex carbohydrates, making foods easier to digest. This can be particularly beneficial for people with digestive issues, such as irritable bowel syndrome (IBS) or lactose intolerance.

2. Boosted Immune System

Gut-Immune Connection:
A significant portion of the immune system is located in the gut. By maintaining a healthy gut microbiome through the consumption of fermented foods, you can enhance your immune response and reduce the risk of infections and illnesses.

Antimicrobial Properties:
Some fermented foods produce natural antimicrobial compounds that can help fight off harmful bacteria and pathogens.

3. Increased Nutrient Availability

Bioavailability:
Fermentation can increase the bioavailability of certain nutrients, making them easier for your body to absorb. For example, the fermentation process

can increase the levels of B vitamins, vitamin K, and minerals like magnesium and zinc.

Nutrient Preservation:
Fermented foods often have a longer shelf life and retain their nutritional value better than non-fermented counterparts.

4. Support for Mental Health

Gut-Brain Axis:
There is a strong connection between the gut and the brain, known as the gut-brain axis. A healthy gut microbiome can positively influence brain function and may help alleviate symptoms of anxiety, depression, and other mental health conditions.

Mood Regulation:
The production of neurotransmitters like serotonin is influenced by gut bacteria. Fermented foods can help promote a healthy balance of these neurotransmitters, supporting mood regulation.

5. Potential Weight Management Benefits

Metabolism Boost:
Probiotics in fermented foods can support a healthy metabolism and aid in weight management by improving digestion and nutrient absorption.

Reduced Inflammation:
Chronic inflammation is linked to weight gain and obesity. Fermented foods can help reduce inflammation in the body, supporting overall metabolic health.

6. Improved Heart Health

Cholesterol Levels:

Some studies suggest that certain probiotics found in fermented foods can help lower LDL (bad) cholesterol levels and increase HDL (good) cholesterol levels, contributing to better heart health.

Blood Pressure:
Fermented foods like kimchi and sauerkraut may also help reduce blood pressure due to their bioactive compounds.

7. Diverse Flavors and Culinary Variety

Enhanced Flavor:
Fermentation can enhance the flavor profile of foods, adding tanginess and depth. This can make healthy eating more enjoyable and sustainable.

Versatility:
Fermented foods come in a variety of forms, including vegetables (kimchi, sauerkraut), dairy (yogurt, kefir), grains (sourdough bread), and beverages (kombucha). This variety allows for creativity in meal planning and cooking.

Examples of Fermented Foods

- **Vegetables**: Kimchi, sauerkraut, pickles (fermented naturally)
- **Dairy:** Yogurt, kefir
- **Grains:** Sourdough bread, tempeh
- **Beverages:** Kombucha, kvass
- **Legumes**: Miso, natto

How to Incorporate Fermented Foods into Your Diet

Start Slowly: If you're new to fermented foods, start with small amounts to allow your digestive system to adjust.
Variety: Incorporate different types of fermented foods to benefit from a range of probiotics and flavors.

Homemade Options: Consider making your own fermented foods at home for better control over ingredients and fermentation processes.
Quality: Choose high-quality, naturally fermented products without added sugars or preservatives.

Including fermented foods in your diet can provide numerous health benefits, making them a valuable addition to a balanced, nutrient-dense eating plan.

More Side Dishes Recipes

Recipe 1: Roasted Brussels Sprouts with Balsamic Glaze

Nutritional Information (per serving):

- Calories: 120
- Protein: 4g
- Carbohydrates: 15g
- Fat: 6g
- Fiber: 6g

Ingredients:

- 1 pound Brussels sprouts, trimmed and halved
- 2 tablespoons olive oil
- Salt to taste
- 2 tablespoons balsamic vinegar
- 1 tablespoon maple syrup (optional)
- Chopped pecans for garnish (optional)

Instructions:

1. Preheat oven to 400°F (200°C).
2. Toss Brussels sprouts with olive oil and salt in a mixing bowl until evenly coated.
3. Spread Brussels sprouts in a single layer on a baking sheet lined with parchment paper.
4. Roast in the preheated oven for 25-30 minutes, or until Brussels sprouts are tender and caramelized, stirring halfway through.
5. In a small saucepan, heat balsamic vinegar and maple syrup (if using) over medium heat until reduced by half and thickened, about 5 minutes.
6. Drizzle the balsamic glaze over the roasted Brussels sprouts before serving.
7. Garnish with chopped pecans if desired.

<u>Dietary Alternatives:</u>

- For low-FODMAP: Omit maple syrup.
- For nut-free: Omit chopped pecans.

<u>Recipe 2: Lemon Garlic Roasted Asparagus</u>

<u>Nutritional Information (per serving):</u>

- Calories: 80
- Protein: 4g
- Carbohydrates: 10g
- Fat: 4g
- Fiber: 4g

<u>Ingredients:</u>

- 1 pound asparagus spears, trimmed
- 2 tablespoons olive oil
- 2 cloves garlic, minced
- Zest of 1 lemon
- Salt to taste
- Lemon wedges for serving (optional)

<u>Instructions:</u>

1. Preheat oven to 400°F (200°C).
2. Toss asparagus spears with olive oil, minced garlic, lemon zest and salt in a mixing bowl until evenly coated.
3. Spread asparagus spears in a single layer on a baking sheet lined with parchment paper.
4. Roast in the preheated oven for 12-15 minutes, or until asparagus is tender and lightly browned, shaking the pan halfway through.
5. Serve hot with lemon wedges on the side if desired.

<u>Dietary Alternatives:</u>

- For low-FODMAP: Omit garlic.
- For garlic-free: Substitute minced garlic with garlic-infused oil.

Recipe 3: Sweet Potato Fries

Nutritional Information (per serving):

- Calories: 150
- Protein: 2g
- Carbohydrates: 30g
- Fat: 4g
- Fiber: 5g

Ingredients:

- 2 large sweet potatoes, peeled and cut into fries
- 2 tablespoons coconut oil, melted
- 1 teaspoon paprika
- 1/2 teaspoon garlic powder
- Salt to taste
- Fresh parsley for garnish (optional)

Instructions:

1. Preheat oven to 425°F (220°C).
2. In a large bowl, toss sweet potato fries with melted coconut oil, paprika, garlic powder and salt, until evenly coated.
3. Spread sweet potato fries in a single layer on a baking sheet lined with parchment paper.
4. Bake in the preheated oven for 20-25 minutes, flipping halfway through, or until fries are crispy and golden brown.
5. Serve hot, garnished with fresh parsley if desired.

Dietary Alternatives:

- For low-FODMAP: Omit garlic powder.
- For nightshade-free: Substitute paprika with smoked paprika or omit it altogether.

Chapter 7:

Desserts and Treats

Mixed Berry Coconut Popsicles

Nutritional Information (per serving):

- Calories: 80
- Protein: 1g
- Carbohydrates: 15g
- Fat: 3g
- Fiber: 5g

Ingredients:

- 1 cup mixed berries (strawberries, blueberries, raspberries)
- 1 can (14 oz) coconut milk
- 2 tablespoons maple syrup (optional)
- 1 teaspoon vanilla extract

Instructions:

1. In a blender, combine mixed berries, coconut milk, maple syrup (if using), and vanilla extract.
2. Blend until smooth.
3. Pour the mixture into popsicle molds.
4. Insert popsicle sticks into the molds.
5. Freeze for at least 4 hours or until solid.
6. To release the popsicles from the molds, run them under warm water for a few seconds.
7. Enjoy these refreshing and nutritious popsicles on a hot day!

Dietary Alternatives:

- For low-sugar: Omit maple syrup or substitute with stevia.
- For coconut-free: Replace coconut milk with almond milk or another non-dairy milk of your choice.

Apple Cinnamon Muffins

Nutritional Information (per serving - 1 muffin):

- Calories: 150
- Protein: 3g
- Carbohydrates: 20g
- Fat: 7g
- Fiber: 3g

Ingredients:

- 2 cups tiger nut flour
- 1 teaspoon baking soda
- 1 teaspoon cinnamon
- 1/4 teaspoon salt
- 2 medium apples, peeled and grated
- 1/4 cup coconut oil, melted
- 1/4 cup maple syrup
- 2 tablespoons coconut milk
- 1 teaspoon vanilla extract

Instructions:

1. Preheat oven to 350°F (175°C). Line a muffin tin with paper liners or grease with coconut oil.
2. In a large mixing bowl, combine tiger nut flour, baking soda, cinnamon, and salt.
3. In another bowl, whisk together grated apples, melted coconut oil, maple syrup, coconut milk, and vanilla extract.
4. Add wet ingredients to dry ingredients and stir until well combined.
5. Spoon the batter into the prepared muffin tin, filling each cup about 3/4 full.
6. Bake for 20-25 minutes or until a toothpick inserted into the center comes out clean.
7. Allow muffins to cool in the pan for 5 minutes, then transfer to a wire rack to cool completely.
8. Enjoy these delicious and moist apple cinnamon muffins as a guilt-free treat!

<u>***Dietary Alternatives:***</u>

- For nut-free: Substitute tiger nut flour with cassava flour or coconut flour.
- For low-FODMAP: Limit the amount of apple used or substitute with mashed banana.

Treats for Special Occasions

<u>Chocolate Avocado Mousse</u>

<u>**Nutritional Information (per serving):**</u>

- Calories: 150
- Protein: 2g
- Carbohydrates: 10g
- Fat: 12g
- Fiber: 5g

<u>**Ingredients:**</u>

- 2 ripe avocados
- 1/4 cup cocoa powder
- 1/4 cup maple syrup or honey
- 1 teaspoon vanilla extract
- Pinch of salt
- Fresh berries for garnish (optional)

<u>Instructions:</u>

1. Scoop the flesh of the avocados into a blender or food processor.
2. Add cocoa powder, maple syrup or honey, vanilla extract, and a pinch of salt.
3. Blend until smooth and creamy, scraping down the sides as needed.
4. Taste and adjust sweetness if necessary by adding more maple syrup or honey.
5. Divide the chocolate avocado mousse into serving cups.
6. Refrigerate for at least 1 hour before serving.
7. Garnish with fresh berries before serving if desired.
8. Enjoy this decadent yet healthy chocolate avocado mousse as a special treat for any occasion!

Dietary Alternatives:

- For low-sugar: Use stevia or another sugar-free sweetener instead of maple syrup or honey.
- For avocado allergies: Substitute avocado with mashed banana or cooked sweet potato.

Desserts and Treats Recipes

Recipe 1: Coconut Flour Banana Bread

Nutritional Information (per serving - 1 slice):

- Calories: 120
- Protein: 3g
- Carbohydrates: 15g
- Fat: 6g
- Fiber: 3g

Ingredients:

- 4 ripe bananas, mashed
- 4 large eggs
- 1/4 cup coconut oil, melted
- 1/4 cup maple syrup or honey
- 1 teaspoon vanilla extract
- 1/2 cup coconut flour
- 1 teaspoon baking soda
- 1/2 teaspoon cinnamon
- Pinch of salt
- Chopped walnuts for garnish (optional)

Instructions:

1. Preheat oven to 350°F (175°C). Grease a loaf pan with coconut oil or line with parchment paper.

2. In a large mixing bowl, whisk together mashed bananas, eggs, melted coconut oil, maple syrup or honey, and vanilla extract until well combined.
3. In a separate bowl, sift together coconut flour, baking soda, cinnamon, and salt.
4. Gradually add the dry ingredients to the wet ingredients, stirring until a smooth batter forms.
5. Pour the batter into the prepared loaf pan and spread evenly.
6. Sprinkle chopped walnuts on top if desired.
7. Bake for 45-50 minutes or until a toothpick inserted into the center comes out clean.
8. Allow banana bread to cool in the pan for 10 minutes, then transfer to a wire rack to cool completely before slicing.
9. Enjoy a slice of this delicious coconut flour banana bread as a wholesome treat any time of the day!

Dietary Alternatives:

- For nut-free: Omit chopped walnuts.
- For low-FODMAP: Limit serving size due to high banana content.

Recipe 2: Lemon Coconut Bliss Balls

Nutritional Information (per serving - 2 balls):

- Calories: 100
- Protein: 2g
- Carbohydrates: 10g
- Fat: 6g
- Fiber: 2g

Ingredients:

- 1 cup shredded coconut, unsweetened
- 1/4 cup coconut butter, softened
- Zest and juice of 1 lemon
- 2 tablespoons maple syrup or honey
- Pinch of salt
- Additional shredded coconut for rolling (optional)

<h1 align="center"><u>Instructions:</u></h1>

1. In a food processor, combine shredded coconut, softened coconut butter, lemon zest, lemon juice, maple syrup or honey, and a pinch of salt.
2. Pulse until the mixture comes together and forms a sticky dough.
3. Roll the dough into small balls, about 1 tablespoon each, using your hands.
4. If desired, roll the balls in additional shredded coconut for coating.
5. Place the bliss balls on a baking sheet lined with parchment paper.
6. Refrigerate for at least 30 minutes to firm up.
7. Once chilled, store the lemon coconut bliss balls in an airtight container in the refrigerator.

Dietary Alternatives:

- For low-sugar: Use stevia or another sugar-free sweetener instead of maple syrup or honey.
- For citrus allergies: Substitute lemon with lime or omit citrus zest and juice altogether.

<h2 align="center"><u>Recipe 3: Berry Crumble Bars</u></h2>

Nutritional Information (per serving - 1 bar):

- Calories: 150
- Protein: 3g
- Carbohydrates: 20g
- Fat: 7g
- Fiber: 5g

Ingredients:

- 2 cups mixed berries (strawberries, blueberries, raspberries)
- 1 tablespoon maple syrup or honey
- 1 tablespoon lemon juice
- 1 cup tiger nut flour
- 1/4 cup coconut oil, melted
- 1/4 cup maple syrup or honey
- 1 teaspoon vanilla extract
- Pinch of salt

<h1 style="text-align:center"><u>Instructions:</u></h1>

1. Preheat oven to 350°F (175°C). Grease an 8x8-inch baking dish with coconut oil or line with parchment paper.
2. In a mixing bowl, toss mixed berries with maple syrup or honey and lemon juice until well coated. Set aside.
3. In another bowl, combine tiger nut flour, melted coconut oil, maple syrup or honey, vanilla extract, and a pinch of salt. Mix until crumbly.
4. Press half of the crumb mixture into the bottom of the prepared baking dish to form the base.
5. Spread the mixed berries evenly over the crumb base.
6. Sprinkle the remaining crumb mixture over the berries as the topping.
7. Bake in the preheated oven for 25-30 minutes or until the top is golden brown and the berries are bubbling.
8. Allow the berry crumble bars to cool completely in the baking dish before slicing into bars.
9. Enjoy these delightful and fruity crumble bars as a delightful dessert or snack!

<u>Dietary Alternatives:</u>

- For low-FODMAP: Limit serving size due to high berry content.
- For nut-free: Substitute tiger nut flour with cassava flour or coconut flour.

Chapter 8:

Beverages

<u>Ginger Turmeric Tea</u>

<u>Nutritional Information (per serving):</u>

- Calories: 10
- Protein: 0g
- Carbohydrates: 3g
- Fat: 0g
- Fiber: 1g

<u>Ingredients:</u>

- 1-inch piece of fresh ginger, sliced
- 1-inch piece of fresh turmeric, sliced (or 1 teaspoon ground turmeric)
- 2 cups water
- 1 tablespoon raw honey (optional)
- Lemon slices for garnish (optional)

<u>Instructions:</u>

1. In a small saucepan, bring water to a boil.
2. Add sliced ginger and turmeric to the boiling water.
3. Reduce heat and let simmer for 5-10 minutes.
4. Remove from heat and strain the tea into mugs.
5. Add raw honey to sweeten if desired.
6. Garnish with lemon slices before serving.

<u>Dietary Alternatives:</u>

- For low-sugar: Omit raw honey or substitute with stevia.
- For citrus allergies: Omit lemon slices.

Smoothies and Juices

Tropical Green Smoothie

Nutritional Information (per serving):

- Calories: 150
- Protein: 3g
- Carbohydrates: 30g
- Fat: 2g
- Fiber: 5g

Ingredients:

- 1 cup fresh spinach
- 1/2 cup frozen mango chunks
- 1/2 cup frozen pineapple chunks
- 1/2 ripe banana
- 1 cup coconut water
- Juice of 1/2 lime
- Ice cubes (optional)

Instructions:

1. Place fresh spinach, frozen mango chunks, frozen pineapple chunks, ripe banana, coconut water, and lime juice in a blender.
2. Blend until smooth and creamy.
3. Add ice cubes if a colder smoothie is desired and blend again.
4. Pour into glasses and serve immediately.
5. Enjoy this refreshing and nutrient-packed tropical green smoothie as a delicious and hydrating snack or breakfast option!

Dietary Alternatives:

- For low-sugar: Use less ripe banana or substitute with stevia.
- For nut-free: Substitute coconut water with water or another non-dairy milk.

Special Occasion Drinks

Watermelon Mint Cooler

Nutritional Information (per serving):

- Calories: 50
- Protein: 1g
- Carbohydrates: 10g
- Fat: 0g
- Fiber: 1g

Ingredients:

- 2 cups seedless watermelon, cubed
- 1/4 cup fresh mint leaves
- 1 tablespoon lime juice
- 1 cup sparkling water
- Ice cubes
- Mint sprigs and watermelon wedges for garnish

Instructions:

1. In a blender, combine seedless watermelon cubes, fresh mint leaves, and lime juice.
2. Blend until smooth.
3. Strain the watermelon mixture through a fine-mesh sieve to remove pulp.
4. Divide the strained watermelon juice into serving glasses filled with ice cubes.
5. Top each glass with sparkling water and gently stir to combine.
6. Garnish with mint sprigs and watermelon wedges.
7. Serve immediately and enjoy this refreshing watermelon mint cooler on a hot day or for a special occasion!

Dietary Alternatives:

- For low-FODMAP: Limit serving size due to high watermelon content.
- For citrus allergies: Omit lime juice or substitute with lemon juice.

More AIP-friendly Beverage Recipes

<h1 style="text-align:center"><u>Recipe 1: Berry Basil Infused Water</u></h1>

<u>Nutritional Information (per serving):</u>

- Calories: 0
- Protein: 0g
- Carbohydrates: 0g
- Fat: 0g
- Fiber: 0g

<u>Ingredients:</u>

- 1 cup mixed berries (strawberries, blueberries, raspberries)
- Handful of fresh basil leaves
- 4 cups filtered water
- Ice cubes

<u>Instructions:</u>

1. In a large pitcher, muddle the mixed berries and basil leaves with a muddler or wooden spoon to release their flavors.
2. Add filtered water to the pitcher and stir to combine.
3. Refrigerate for at least 1 hour to allow the flavors to infuse.
4. Serve the berry basil infused water over ice cubes.
5. Enjoy this refreshing and hydrating beverage as a delightful alternative to plain water!

<u>Dietary Alternatives:</u>

- For low-FODMAP: Limit serving size due to high berry content.
- For herb allergies: Omit basil leaves or substitute with mint leaves.

<h1 style="text-align:center"><u>Recipe 2: Turmeric Coconut Latte</u></h1>

Nutritional Information (per serving):

- Calories: 100
- Protein: 1g
- Carbohydrates: 5g
- Fat: 9g
- Fiber: 1g

Ingredients:

- 1 cup coconut milk
- 1 teaspoon ground turmeric
- 1/2 teaspoon ground cinnamon
- Pinch of ground ginger
- Pinch of black pepper
- 1 tablespoon maple syrup or honey (optional)

Instructions:

1. In a small saucepan, heat coconut milk over medium heat until hot but not boiling.
2. Whisk in ground turmeric, ground cinnamon, ground ginger, and black pepper until well combined.
3. Stir in maple syrup or honey if using, and continue to heat until the latte is steaming.
4. Pour the turmeric coconut latte into mugs and serve immediately.
5. Enjoy this comforting and immune-boosting beverage as a soothing treat any time of the day!

Dietary Alternatives:

- For low-sugar: Omit maple syrup or honey or substitute with stevia.
- For nut-free: Substitute coconut milk with another non-dairy milk.

Recipe 3: Pineapple Mint Sparkler

Nutritional Information (per serving):

- Calories: 80
- Protein: 0g
- Carbohydrates: 20g
- Fat: 0g
- Fiber: 1g

Ingredients:

- 1 cup fresh pineapple chunks
- Handful of fresh mint leaves
- 1 tablespoon lime juice
- 2 cups sparkling water
- Ice cubes
- Pineapple wedges and mint sprigs for garnish

Instructions:

1. In a blender, combine fresh pineapple chunks, fresh mint leaves, and lime juice.
2. Blend until smooth.
3. Strain the pineapple mint mixture through a fine-mesh sieve to remove pulp.
4. Divide the strained mixture into serving glasses filled with ice cubes.
5. Top each glass with sparkling water and gently stir to combine.
6. Garnish with pineapple wedges and mint sprigs.
7. Serve immediately and enjoy this tropical and refreshing pineapple mint sparkler as a delightful mocktail!

Dietary Alternatives:

- For low-FODMAP: Limit serving size due to high pineapple content.
- For citrus allergies: Omit lime juice or substitute with lemon juice.

Chapter 9:

Special Occasions and Entertaining

Holiday Recipes

Roast Turkey with Cranberry Sauce

Nutritional Information (per serving - turkey with sauce):	Ingredients for Turkey:	Ingredients for Cranberry Sauce:
• Calories: 300 • Protein: 30g • Carbohydrates: 15g • Fat: 12g • Fiber: 2g	• 1 whole turkey (10-12 pounds), thawed if frozen • 1/4 cup olive oil • Salt taste	• 2 cups fresh cranberries • 1/2 cup orange juice • 1/4 cup maple syrup • 1 teaspoon grated orange zest

Instructions for Turkey:

1. Preheat oven to 325°F (165°C).
2. Remove giblets from the turkey cavity and pat dry with paper towels.
3. Rub olive oil over the turkey skin and season generously with salt.
4. Place the turkey on a roasting rack in a roasting pan breast side up.
5. Roast the turkey in the preheated oven for 3 to 3 1/2 hours, or until the internal temperature reaches 165°F (75°C) in the thickest part of the thigh.
6. Remove the turkey from the oven and let it rest for 20 minutes before carving.

<u>**Instructions for Cranberry Sauce:**</u>

1. In a saucepan, combine fresh cranberries, orange juice, maple syrup, and orange zest.
2. Bring to a boil over medium heat, then reduce heat and simmer for 10-15 minutes, or until cranberries burst and sauce thickens.
3. Remove from heat and let cool before serving with roast turkey.

<u>*Dietary Alternatives:*</u>

- For low-sugar: Use stevia instead of maple syrup in cranberry sauce.
- For citrus allergies: Omit orange zest and use water instead of orange juice in cranberry sauce.

<u>Party Appetizers and Finger Foods</u>

<u>Bacon-Wrapped Dates with Herbed Cashew Cheese</u>

<u>Nutritional Information (per serving - 2 pieces):</u>

- Calories: 120
- Protein: 3g
- Carbohydrates: 8g
- Fat: 9g
- Fiber: 1g

<u>Ingredients:</u>

- 12 Medjool dates, pitted
- 6 slices bacon, cut in half crosswise
- 1/2 cup cashews, soaked for 2 hours and drained
- 2 tablespoons coconut milk
- 1 tablespoon lemon juice
- 1 tablespoon chopped fresh herbs (such as parsley, thyme, or rosemary)
- Salt to taste

Instructions:

1. Preheat oven to 375°F (190°C).
2. Slice each date lengthwise and remove the pit.
3. In a food processor, combine soaked cashews, coconut milk, lemon juice, chopped herbs and salt. Blend until smooth to make the herbed cashew cheese.
4. Stuff each date with a small spoonful of herbed cashew cheese.
5. Wrap each stuffed date with a half slice of bacon and secure with a toothpick.
6. Place the bacon-wrapped dates on a baking sheet lined with parchment paper.
7. Bake in the preheated oven for 15-20 minutes, or until the bacon is crispy.
8. Remove from the oven and let cool slightly before serving.

Dietary Alternatives:

- For nut-free: Use coconut cream instead of cashews for the cheese filling.
- For pork-free: Substitute bacon with turkey bacon or prosciutto.

Entertaining Tips

- **Plan Ahead:** Plan your menu and shopping list in advance to ensure you have all the ingredients you need for your celebration meals.
- **Prep in Advance:** Prepare dishes that can be made ahead of time and reheated before serving to reduce stress on the day of the event.
- **Consider Dietary Restrictions:** Take into account any dietary restrictions or preferences of your guests and offer a variety of options to accommodate everyone.
- **Decorate Thoughtfully**: Add festive decorations and table settings to create a welcoming atmosphere for your guests.

More AIP-friendly Recipes for Special Occasions

Recipe 1: Herb-Crusted Roast Beef

Nutritional Information (per serving):

- Calories: 250
- Protein: 30g
- Carbohydrates: 0g
- Fat: 14g
- Fiber: 0g

Ingredients:

- 2 pounds beef roast (such as sirloin or ribeye)
- 2 tablespoons chopped fresh herbs (such as rosemary, thyme, and sage)
- 2 cloves garlic, minced
- 2 tablespoons olive oil
- Salt to taste

Instructions:

1. Preheat oven to 375°F (190°C).
2. In a small bowl, mix together chopped fresh herbs, minced garlic, olive oil and salt to make the herb crust.
3. Rub the herb crust mixture all over the beef roast, covering it evenly.
4. Place the seasoned beef roast on a roasting rack in a roasting pan.
5. Roast in the preheated oven for about 1 hour, or until the internal temperature reaches your desired level of doneness (135°F for medium-rare, 145°F for medium).
6. Remove the roast from the oven and let it rest for 10 minutes before slicing.
7. Slice the roast beef thinly and serve with your favorite AIP-friendly side dishes.

Dietary Alternatives:

- For herb allergies: Omit fresh herbs or substitute with dried herbs.
- For low-FODMAP: Limit garlic or use garlic-infused oil.

<h1 align="center"><u>Recipe 2: Stuffed Acorn Squash with Ground Turkey</u></h1>

<u>Nutritional Information (per serving):</u>

- Calories: 200
- Protein: 15g
- Carbohydrates: 20g
- Fat: 8g
- Fiber: 5g

<u>Ingredients:</u>

- 2 acorn squash, halved and seeds removed
- 1 pound ground turkey
- 1 onion, diced
- 2 cloves garlic, minced
- 1 teaspoon ground sage
- 1 teaspoon ground cinnamon
- Salt to taste
- 1 tablespoon olive oil
- Fresh parsley for garnish (optional)

<u>Instructions:</u>

1. Preheat oven to 375°F (190°C).
2. Place acorn squash halves cut side down on a baking sheet lined with parchment paper. Bake for 30 minutes, or until tender.
3. In a skillet, heat olive oil over medium heat. Add diced onion and minced garlic, and sauté until softened.
4. Add ground turkey to the skillet and cook until browned, breaking it up with a spoon as it cooks.
5. Stir in ground sage, ground cinnamon, salt, and pepper (if tolerated).
6. Once the turkey is cooked through, remove from heat.
7. Once the acorn squash halves are tender, remove them from the oven and flip them over.
8. Fill each acorn squash half with the cooked ground turkey mixture.
9. Return the stuffed squash to the oven and bake for an additional 15 minutes.
10. Garnish with fresh parsley before serving, if desired.

- For low-FODMAP: Omit onion or use green onion tops instead.
- For nightshade allergies: Omit ground pepper or substitute with other AIP-friendly seasonings.

Recipe 3: Lemon Herb Grilled Chicken Skewers

Nutritional Information (per serving):

- Calories: 180
- Protein: 25g
- Carbohydrates: 2g
- Fat: 8g
- Fiber: 0g

Ingredients:

- 1 pound boneless, skinless chicken breasts, cut into cubes
- Zest and juice of 1 lemon
- 2 tablespoons chopped fresh herbs (such as rosemary, thyme, and parsley)
- 2 cloves garlic, minced
- 2 tablespoons olive oil
- Salt and pepper (if tolerated) to taste
- Wooden skewers, soaked in water for 30 minutes

Instructions:

1. In a bowl, combine lemon zest, lemon juice, chopped fresh herbs, minced garlic, olive oil, salt, and pepper to make the marinade.
2. Add the chicken cubes to the marinade and toss to coat evenly. Cover and refrigerate for at least 30 minutes, or up to 4 hours.
3. Preheat grill or grill pan over medium-high heat.
4. Thread marinated chicken cubes onto wooden skewers.

5. Grill the chicken skewers for 5-7 minutes on each side, or until cooked through and lightly charred.
6. Remove from grill and let rest for a few minutes before serving.
7. Serve the lemon herb grilled chicken skewers with your favorite AIP-friendly side dishes.

Dietary Alternatives:

- For low-FODMAP: Omit garlic or use garlic-infused oil.
- For citrus allergies: Omit lemon zest and juice or substitute with apple cider vinegar.

Chapter 10:

Lifestyle and Long-Term Success

In this final chapter, we will talk about how to adapt to the Autoimmune Protocol (AIP) lifestyle for long-term success. Navigating social situations, dining out, and traveling while on the AIP can present challenges, but with the right strategies, you can maintain your health goals and enjoy life to the fullest.

1. Adapting to the AIP Lifestyle

Living the AIP lifestyle involves more than just following a specific diet—it's about embracing a holistic approach to wellness that encompasses your physical, mental, and emotional well-being. Here are some tips to help you navigate various aspects of life while on the AIP:

Tips for Dining Out

- **Plan Ahead:** Research restaurants that offer AIP-friendly options and review their menus online before dining out.
- **Communicate Clearly:** When ordering, communicate your dietary restrictions to your server and ask questions about ingredients and preparation methods.
- **Customize Your Order:** Don't hesitate to ask for modifications to menu items to make them AIP-compliant, such as requesting grilled instead of fried or asking for sauces and dressings on the side.
- **Be Flexible:** In some situations, you may need to make compromises or adjustments to your meal, but remember that progress, not perfection, is key.

Managing Social Situations

- **Educate Others:** Take the opportunity to educate friends and family about the AIP and why it's important for managing your autoimmune condition.

- **Offer to Contribute:** When attending social gatherings or potlucks, offer to bring AIP-friendly dishes to ensure there are options available that you can enjoy.
- **Focus on Connections:** While food is often a central aspect of social gatherings, remember that the true purpose is to connect with others. Shift the focus away from food and onto meaningful conversations and activities.

Traveling While on AIP

- **Pack Snacks:** Bring AIP-friendly snacks with you when traveling to avoid getting hungry and tempted by non-compliant foods.
- **Research Local Options:** Look up restaurants and grocery stores at your destination that offer AIP-friendly options or ingredients.
- **Stay Flexible:** While it's ideal to stick to your AIP plan as much as possible, be prepared to make adjustments and choose the best available options when traveling.

2. Mental and Emotional Well-being

Adopting the Autoimmune Protocol (AIP) diet is not just about what you eat—it's also about nurturing your mental and emotional health. Stress management, mindfulness, and having a strong support network are crucial components of your overall well-being. Let's explore these aspects in detail to help you achieve a balanced and fulfilling lifestyle.

Stress Management Techniques

Chronic stress can exacerbate autoimmune conditions, making it essential to incorporate stress management techniques into your daily routine. Here are some effective methods:

- **Deep Breathing Exercises:** Simple breathing exercises can help calm your nervous system. Try inhaling deeply for four counts, holding for four counts, and exhaling for four counts. Repeat several times.

- **Physical Activity:** Engage in gentle exercises like walking, yoga, or tai chi. Physical activity releases endorphins, which can improve your mood and reduce stress.
- **Hobbies and Interests:** Spend time on activities that you enjoy, whether it's reading, gardening, painting, or any other hobby. Doing things you love can provide a much-needed mental break.

Mindfulness and Meditation

Mindfulness and meditation can significantly enhance your mental and emotional well-being. These practices help you stay present, reduce anxiety, and improve your overall mood.

- **Mindfulness Practices:** Being mindful means paying full attention to the present moment. You can practice mindfulness by focusing on your breath, observing your surroundings, or savoring each bite of your meal.
- **Meditation**: Regular meditation can help calm your mind and reduce stress. Start with just a few minutes each day. Find a quiet space, sit comfortably, and focus on your breath. Guided meditations can also be helpful.
- **Gratitude Journaling:** Keep a journal where you write down things you're grateful for each day. This practice can shift your focus from stressors to positive aspects of your life, promoting a more positive mindset.

Support Networks and Resources

Having a strong support network is invaluable when managing an autoimmune condition and adhering to the AIP diet. Connecting with others who understand your journey can provide emotional support and practical advice.

- **Family and Friends:** Share your experiences and challenges with your loved ones. They can offer support, encouragement, and even help with meal preparation.

- **Online Communities:** Join online forums and social media groups dedicated to the AIP lifestyle. These communities can provide a wealth of information, recipe ideas, and moral support.
- **Support Groups:** Look for local or virtual support groups where you can meet others dealing with similar health issues. Sharing your experiences and hearing from others can be incredibly reassuring.
- **Professional Help:** Don't hesitate to seek professional support if needed. A therapist or counselor can help you navigate emotional challenges, while a nutritionist can offer guidance on the AIP diet.

Final Thoughts

Caring for your mental and emotional well-being is just as important as managing your diet when it comes to the AIP lifestyle. By engaging in stress management techniques, practicing mindfulness and meditation, and building a strong support network, you can create a holistic approach to health that nurtures both your body and mind.

Remember, the journey to better health is a marathon, not a sprint. Celebrate your progress, be kind to yourself, and use these tools to maintain a balanced and fulfilling life while following the AIP diet.

Conclusion

1. Words of Encouragement

As we come to the end of this AIP Diet Cookbook, I want to leave you with a few words of encouragement and motivation. Your journey to better health through the Autoimmune Protocol (AIP) is a significant and commendable step towards a healthier, happier life.

Motivational Message for Readers

Embarking on the AIP journey is no small feat. It requires dedication, patience, and a willingness to make meaningful changes to your lifestyle. But remember, every small step you take towards better health is a victory. Celebrate your successes, no matter how small they may seem. Each meal you prepare, each time you choose an AIP-friendly option, you are making a positive impact on your health and well-being.

Your commitment to the AIP diet is an investment in yourself. It's a declaration that you value your health and are willing to put in the effort to feel better. There will be challenges along the way, and that's okay. It's all part of the process. Embrace these challenges as opportunities to learn and grow. Over time, you will find that these efforts become second nature, and the benefits you reap will make it all worthwhile.

Encouragement to Personalize and Adapt the Diet

One of the most empowering aspects of the AIP is its flexibility. While there are general guidelines to follow, it's important to remember that everyone's journey is unique. What works for one person might not work for another, and that's perfectly okay. Take the time to listen to your body and understand its needs.

Feel free to personalize and adapt the AIP diet to suit your lifestyle and preferences. Experiment with different recipes, ingredients, and cooking methods to find what works best for you. Don't be afraid to make modifications based on your individual health requirements and taste preferences. The goal is to create a sustainable and enjoyable way of eating that supports your health.

Remember, the AIP is not just a diet—it's a holistic approach to wellness that includes not only what you eat but also how you manage stress, sleep, and exercise. Integrate these elements into your life in a way that feels right for you.

In conclusion, know that you are not alone on this journey. There is a community of people who understand what you are going through and are there to support you. Keep moving forward, stay positive, and believe in your ability to create a healthier, more vibrant life. You've got this!

As you close this book, take with you the knowledge, recipes, and tips you've gained, and use them as tools to build a healthier future. Your dedication and effort are commendable, and I wish you all the success and well-being in your AIP journey. Thank you for allowing this cookbook to be a part of your path to better health.

Appendices

1. AIP Food Lists

Comprehensive Lists of Approved and Eliminated Foods

Approved Foods:

- **Vegetables:** Leafy greens (kale, spinach), cruciferous vegetables (broccoli, cauliflower), root vegetables (sweet potatoes, carrots), squashes (butternut, acorn), sea vegetables (nori, kelp)
- **Fruits:** Berries (blueberries, strawberries), apples, bananas, citrus fruits (oranges, lemons), melons (watermelon, cantaloupe), tropical fruits (mango, papaya)
- **Meats and Seafood:** Grass-fed beef, pasture-raised poultry, wild-caught fish (salmon, cod), shellfish (shrimp, crab), organ meats (liver, heart)
- **Fats:** Olive oil, coconut oil, avocado oil, lard, tallow
- **Herbs and Spices:** Basil, oregano, thyme, rosemary, turmeric, ginger
- **Beverages:** Herbal teas (chamomile, peppermint), bone broth, coconut water
- **Others:** Coconut milk, coconut flour, cassava flour, arrowroot starch

Eliminated Foods:

- **Grains:** Wheat, rice, oats, corn, quinoa, barley
- **Dairy:** Milk, cheese, yogurt, butter
- **Legumes:** Beans, lentils, peanuts, soy products
- **Nuts and Seeds:** Almonds, cashews, chia seeds, sunflower seeds
- **Nightshades:** Tomatoes, potatoes, eggplants, bell peppers
- **Processed Foods:** Sugary snacks, soda, packaged snacks with additives
- **Additives:** Artificial sweeteners, preservatives, food colorings

2. Shopping Lists

Sample Grocery Lists for Different Phases of AIP

Elimination Phase:

- **Vegetables:** Kale, spinach, broccoli, cauliflower, sweet potatoes, carrots, butternut squash, nori sheets
- **Fruits:** Blueberries, apples, bananas, oranges
- **Proteins:** Grass-fed beef, pasture-raised chicken, wild-caught salmon, shrimp, beef liver
- **Fats:** Olive oil, coconut oil, avocado oil
- **Herbs and Spices**: Basil, oregano, turmeric, ginger
- **Others:** Coconut milk, coconut flour, cassava flour, bone broth

Reintroduction Phase:

- **Vegetables:** All from the elimination phase plus white potatoes (if tolerated)
- **Fruits:** All from the elimination phase plus cherries and peaches (if tolerated)
- **Proteins:** All from the elimination phase plus pasture-raised pork (if tolerated)
- **Fats:** All from the elimination phase plus ghee (if tolerated)
- **Herbs and Spices:** All from the elimination phase plus black pepper (if tolerated)
- **Others:** All from the elimination phase plus dark chocolate (if tolerated)

4-Week AIP-Friendly Meal Plan

Below is a comprehensive 4-week meal plan designed to help you get started on the Autoimmune Protocol (AIP) diet. This plan includes a variety of nutrient-dense, AIP-friendly recipes for breakfast, lunch, dinner, and snacks. Each week is balanced to ensure you get a mix of proteins, vegetables, and healthy fats.

NOTE: The meal plans are just sample plans. You can switch the meals to suit your personal requirements.

WEEKLY MEAL PLAN

WEEK 1

	BREAKFAST	LUNCH	DINNER	SNACKS
MON	SWEET POTATO HASH WITH GROUND TURKEY AND SPINACH	CHICKEN AND VEGETABLE SOUP WITH BONE BROTH	BAKED SALMON WITH ROASTED BRUSSELS SPROUTS AND MASHED CAULIFLOWER	APPLE SLICES WITH COCONUT BUTTER, CARROT STICKS WITH GUACAMOLE
TUE	BERRY SMOOTHIE WITH COCONUT MILK AND SPINACH	MIXED GREENS SALAD WITH GRILLED CHICKEN, AVOCADO, AND OLIVE OIL DRESSING	BEEF STEW WITH ROOT VEGETABLES AND BONE BROTH	BANANA WITH COCONUT FLAKES, CUCUMBER SLICES WITH AIP-FRIENDLY HUMMUS
WED	WARM COCONUT PORRIDGE WITH BLUEBERRIES AND CINNAMON	TURKEY LETTUCE WRAPS WITH AVOCADO AND CUCUMBER	HERB-CRUSTED ROAST BEEF WITH GARLIC MASHED CAULIFLOWER AND STEAMED BROCCOLI	BAKED APPLE WITH COCONUT CRUMBLE, CELERY STICKS WITH LIVER PÂTÉ
THU	MANGO SMOOTHIE BOWL WITH COCONUT MILK AND SPINACH	ASPARAGUS AND CHICKEN SALAD WITH LEMON VINAIGRETTE	GRILLED FISH WITH SPRING VEGETABLES (ARTICHOKES, PEAS)	STRAWBERRIES WITH COCONUT WHIPPED CREAM, RADISHES WITH AVOCADO DIP
FRI	SWEET POTATO AND APPLE HASH WITH GROUND PORK	BUTTERNUT SQUASH SOUP WITH GROUND TURKEY	BRAISED LAMB WITH ROOT VEGETABLE MASH	ORANGE SLICES WITH COCONUT CHIPS, BELL PEPPER SLICES WITH GUACAMOLE
SAT	GREEN SMOOTHIE WITH KALE, BANANA, AND COCONUT MILK	CHICKEN SALAD WITH MIXED GREENS, CUCUMBER, AND OLIVE OIL	PORK CHOPS WITH ROASTED SWEET POTATOES AND SAUTÉED SPINACH	PEAR SLICES WITH COCONUT BUTTER, CUCUMBER SLICES WITH TUNA SALAD
SUN	WARM COCONUT PORRIDGE WITH SLICED BANANA AND CINNAMON	SHRIMP AND AVOCADO SALAD WITH MIXED GREENS	BEEF AND VEGETABLE STIR-FRY WITH CAULIFLOWER RICE	BLUEBERRIES WITH COCONUT WHIPPED CREAM, CARROT STICKS WITH AIP-FRIENDLY HUMMUS

WEEKLY MEAL PLAN

WEEK 2

	BREAKFAST	LUNCH	DINNER	SNACKS
MON	COCONUT YOGURT WITH FRESH BERRIES	GRILLED CHICKEN WITH MIXED GREENS AND AVOCADO	LEMON HERB CHICKEN WITH ROASTED CARROTS AND PARSNIPS	APPLE SLICES WITH SUNFLOWER SEED BUTTER, CUCUMBER STICKS WITH AIP-FRIENDLY HUMMUS
TUE	BUTTERNUT SQUASH BREAKFAST BAKE	SHRIMP AND MANGO SALAD WITH LIME DRESSING	BEEF AND BROCCOLI STIR-FRY WITH CAULIFLOWER RICE	SLICED PEAR WITH COCONUT CHIPS, CARROT STICKS WITH GUACAMOLE
WED	PUMPKIN SMOOTHIE WITH COCONUT MILK AND SPINACH	TURKEY AND SWEET POTATO PATTIES WITH MIXED GREENS	HERB-CRUSTED PORK TENDERLOIN WITH GARLIC MASHED PARSNIPS	BLUEBERRIES WITH COCONUT WHIPPED CREAM, RADISH SLICES WITH AVOCADO DIP
THU	AIP-FRIENDLY PANCAKES WITH BLUEBERRIES	CHICKEN AND AVOCADO LETTUCE WRAPS	LAMB STEW WITH ROOT VEGETABLES	STRAWBERRIES WITH COCONUT FLAKES, CELERY STICKS WITH SUNFLOWER SEED BUTTER
FRI	APPLE-CINNAMON COCONUT PORRIDGE	SALMON AND AVOCADO SALAD WITH LEMON VINAIGRETTE	BAKED COD WITH ZUCCHINI NOODLES AND PESTO	ORANGE SLICES WITH COCONUT CHIPS, BELL PEPPER SLICES WITH AIP-FRIENDLY HUMMUS
SAT	BANANA-COCONUT SMOOTHIE WITH SPINACH	TURKEY AND CRANBERRY SALAD WITH MIXED GREENS	GINGER-GARLIC SHRIMP WITH STEAMED ASPARAGUS	GRAPES WITH COCONUT BUTTER, CUCUMBER SLICES WITH TUNA SALAD
SUN	SWEET POTATO BREAKFAST HASH WITH SAUSAGE	BEEF AND AVOCADO LETTUCE WRAPS	ROASTED CHICKEN THIGHS WITH BRUSSELS SPROUTS AND CAULIFLOWER MASH	PEAR SLICES WITH SUNFLOWER SEED BUTTER, CARROT STICKS WITH GUACAMOLE

WEEKLY MEAL PLAN

WEEK 3

	BREAKFAST	LUNCH	DINNER	SNACKS
MON	COCONUT YOGURT WITH MANGO AND CHIA-FREE GRANOLA	GRILLED CHICKEN SALAD WITH ARUGULA AND STRAWBERRIES	LEMON DILL SALMON WITH ROASTED BEETS AND KALE	APPLE SLICES WITH COCONUT BUTTER, CELERY STICKS WITH LIVER PÂTÉ
TUE	AIP-FRIENDLY SMOOTHIE BOWL WITH SPINACH AND BERRIES	SHRIMP AND AVOCADO LETTUCE WRAPS	BEEF AND VEGETABLE SKEWERS WITH SWEET POTATO WEDGES	BANANA WITH COCONUT FLAKES, CUCUMBER STICKS WITH AIP-FRIENDLY HUMMUS
WED	PUMPKIN BREAKFAST BAKE WITH SPINACH	TURKEY AND APPLE SALAD WITH MIXED GREENS	HERB-ROASTED PORK CHOPS WITH ROASTED ROOT VEGETABLES	BLUEBERRIES WITH COCONUT WHIPPED CREAM, RADISH SLICES WITH AVOCADO DIP
THU	BUTTERNUT SQUASH PORRIDGE WITH CINNAMON	CHICKEN SALAD WITH GRAPES AND WALNUTS	GINGER-LIME SHRIMP WITH CAULIFLOWER FRIED RICE	STRAWBERRIES WITH COCONUT FLAKES, CARROT STICKS WITH GUACAMOLE
FRI	AIP-FRIENDLY PANCAKES WITH APPLE COMPOTE	SALMON SALAD WITH SPINACH AND CUCUMBER	SLOW-COOKED LAMB SHANKS WITH CARROT MASH	ORANGE SLICES WITH COCONUT CHIPS, BELL PEPPER SLICES WITH AIP-FRIENDLY HUMMUS
SAT	BANANA-COCONUT SMOOTHIE WITH KALE	TURKEY AND CRANBERRY LETTUCE WRAPS	BAKED MAHI MAHI WITH ZUCCHINI NOODLES AND TOMATO SAUCE	GRAPES WITH COCONUT BUTTER, CUCUMBER SLICES WITH TUNA SALAD
SUN	SWEET POTATO BREAKFAST HASH WITH GROUND TURKEY	BEEF AND AVOCADO SALAD WITH MIXED GREENS	ROASTED CHICKEN DRUMSTICKS WITH BROCCOLI AND CAULIFLOWER MASH	PEAR SLICES WITH SUNFLOWER SEED BUTTER, CARROT STICKS WITH GUACAMOLE

WEEKLY MEAL PLAN

WEEK 4

	BREAKFAST	LUNCH	DINNER	SNACKS
MON	BLUEBERRY COCONUT SMOOTHIE	CHICKEN ZOODLE SOUP	SLOW-COOKED BEEF WITH MASHED BUTTERNUT SQUASH	APPLE SLICES WITH COCONUT BUTTER, CARROT STICKS WITH AIP-FRIENDLY RANCH
TUE	PLANTAIN AND BACON HASH	AVOCADO CHICKEN SALAD WITH MIXED GREENS	LEMON GARLIC SHRIMP WITH SAUTÉED SPINACH	SLICED PEAR WITH COCONUT FLAKES, CUCUMBER STICKS WITH GUACAMOLE
WED	COCONUT YOGURT WITH MIXED BERRIES AND HONEY	TURKEY MEATBALLS WITH ZUCCHINI NOODLES	HERB-CRUSTED LAMB CHOPS WITH ROASTED VEGETABLES	BLUEBERRIES WITH COCONUT WHIPPED CREAM, RADISH SLICES WITH AVOCADO DIP
THU	SWEET POTATO AND APPLE BAKE	GRILLED SALMON SALAD WITH CUCUMBER AND AVOCADO	BALSAMIC GLAZED CHICKEN WITH ROASTED BRUSSELS SPROUTS	STRAWBERRIES WITH COCONUT CHIPS, CELERY STICKS WITH SUNFLOWER SEED BUTTER
FRI	TROPICAL GREEN SMOOTHIE WITH SPINACH AND PINEAPPLE	BEEF LETTUCE WRAPS WITH AVOCADO AND CUCUMBER	ROASTED PORK TENDERLOIN WITH SWEET POTATO MASH AND STEAMED BROCCOLI	ORANGE SLICES WITH COCONUT CHIPS, BELL PEPPER SLICES WITH AIP-FRIENDLY HUMMUS
SAT	WARM BANANA-COCONUT PORRIDGE	SHRIMP AND AVOCADO SALAD WITH MANGO DRESSING	GARLIC HERB ROASTED CHICKEN WITH CAULIFLOWER RICE	GRAPES WITH COCONUT BUTTER, CUCUMBER SLICES WITH TUNA SALAD
SUN	PUMPKIN AND SPINACH SMOOTHIE	TURKEY AND CRANBERRY LETTUCE WRAPS	GRILLED LAMB KEBABS WITH ROASTED ROOT VEGETABLES	PEAR SLICES WITH SUNFLOWER SEED BUTTER, CARROT STICKS WITH GUACAMOLE

Recipes for Some Featured Dishes

Sweet Potato Hash with Ground Turkey and Spinach:

- **Ingredients**:
    1. 2 medium sweet potatoes, diced
    2. 1 pound ground turkey
    3. 2 cups fresh spinach
    4. 1 tablespoon coconut oil
    5. Salt and pepper to taste
- **Instructions**:
    1. Heat coconut oil in a large skillet over medium heat.
    2. Add diced sweet potatoes and cook until tender, about 10-15 minutes.
    3. Add ground turkey and cook until browned.
    4. Add spinach and cook until wilted.
    5. Season with salt and pepper to taste.

Baked Salmon with Roasted Brussels Sprouts and Mashed Cauliflower:

- **Ingredients:**
    1. 4 salmon fillets
    2. 1 pound Brussels sprouts, halved
    3. 1 large cauliflower head, chopped
    4. 2 tablespoons olive oil
    5. Salt and pepper (if tolerated) to taste
- **Instructions:**
    1. Preheat oven to 400°F (200°C).
    2. Toss Brussels sprouts with 1 tablespoon olive oil, salt, and pepper. Spread on a baking sheet.
    3. Place salmon fillets on another baking sheet, drizzle with remaining olive oil, and season with salt and pepper.

4. Roast Brussels sprouts and salmon for 20 minutes, until sprouts are crispy and salmon is cooked through.
5. Meanwhile, steam cauliflower until tender, then mash with a fork or blender until smooth. Season with salt and pepper.

Warm Coconut Porridge with Blueberries and Cinnamon:

- **Ingredients:**
    1. 1/2 cup coconut milk
    2. 1/2 cup water
    3. 1/4 cup coconut flour
    4. 1/2 cup fresh blueberries
    5. 1/2 teaspoon cinnamon
    6. 1 tablespoon honey (optional)
- **Instructions:**
    1. In a small pot, combine coconut milk, water, and coconut flour.
    2. Cook over medium heat, stirring constantly until thickened, about 5-7 minutes.
    3. Remove from heat and stir in blueberries and cinnamon.
    4. Sweeten with honey if desired.

Butternut Squash Breakfast Bake:

Ingredients:
- 1 medium butternut squash, peeled and diced
- 1 pound ground turkey
- 2 cups fresh spinach
- 1 tablespoon coconut oil
- Salt to taste

Instructions:
1. Preheat oven to 375°F (190°C).
2. Heat coconut oil in a skillet over medium heat.
3. Add ground turkey and cook until browned.

4. Add butternut squash and cook until tender.
5. Add spinach and cook until wilted.
6. Transfer mixture to a baking dish and bake for 20 minutes.

Lemon Herb Chicken with Roasted Carrots and Parsnips:

Ingredients:
- 4 chicken breasts
- 4 large carrots, peeled and sliced
- 4 large parsnips, peeled and sliced
- 2 tablespoons olive oil
- Juice of 1 lemon
- 1 tablespoon fresh thyme leaves
- Salt to taste

Instructions:
1. Preheat oven to 400°F (200°C).
2. Toss carrots and parsnips with 1 tablespoon olive oil and salt. Spread on a baking sheet.
3. Place chicken breasts on another baking sheet, drizzle with remaining olive oil, lemon juice, and thyme. Season with salt and pepper.
4. Roast vegetables and chicken for 25-30 minutes, until vegetables are tender and chicken is cooked through.

Pumpkin Smoothie with Coconut Milk and Spinach:

Ingredients:
- 1 cup pumpkin puree
- 1 cup coconut milk
- 1 cup fresh spinach
- 1 banana
- 1 teaspoon cinnamon

Instructions:
1. Combine all ingredients in a blender.
2. Blend until smooth.

3. Serve immediately.

Herb-Crusted Pork Tenderloin with Garlic Mashed Parsnips:

Ingredients:
- 1 pork tenderloin
- 2 tablespoons olive oil
- 2 tablespoons fresh rosemary, chopped
- 4 large parsnips, peeled and chopped
- 2 garlic cloves, minced
- Salt to taste

Instructions:
1. Preheat oven to 375°F (190°C).
2. Rub pork tenderloin with olive oil, rosemary, and salt.
3. Place on a baking sheet and roast for 25-30 minutes.
4. Meanwhile, boil parsnips until tender. Drain and mash with garlic, salt, and pepper.

Butternut Squash Breakfast Bake:

Ingredients:
- 1 medium butternut squash, peeled and diced
- 1 pound ground turkey
- 2 cups fresh spinach
- 1 tablespoon coconut oil
- Salt and pepper to taste

Instructions:
1. Preheat oven to 375°F (190°C).
2. Heat coconut oil in a skillet over medium heat.
3. Add ground turkey and cook until browned.
4. Add butternut squash and cook until tender.
5. Add spinach and cook until wilted.
6. Transfer mixture to a baking dish and bake for 20 minutes.

Lemon Herb Chicken with Roasted Carrots and Parsnips:

Ingredients:
- 4 chicken breasts
- 4 large carrots, peeled and sliced
- 4 large parsnips, peeled and sliced
- 2 tablespoons olive oil
- Juice of 1 lemon
- 1 tablespoon fresh thyme leaves
- Salt to taste

Instructions:
1. Preheat oven to 400°F (200°C).
2. Toss carrots and parsnips with 1 tablespoon olive oil and salt. Spread on a baking sheet.
3. Place chicken breasts on another baking sheet, drizzle with remaining olive oil, lemon juice, and thyme. Season with salt and pepper.
4. Roast vegetables and chicken for 25-30 minutes, until vegetables are tender and chicken is cooked through.

Pumpkin Smoothie with Coconut Milk and Spinach:

Ingredients:
- 1 cup pumpkin puree
- 1 cup coconut milk
- 1 cup fresh spinach
- 1 banana
- 1 teaspoon cinnamon

Instructions:
1. Combine all ingredients in a blender.
2. Blend until smooth.
3. Serve immediately.